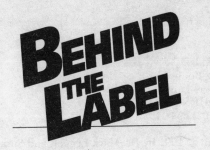

Published by
Schwartz Books
45 Flinders Lane
MELBOURNE 3000
Phone: (03) 654 6433

National Library of Australia
Cataloguing-in-Publication entry

Dr. Mark Leggett and Susan Leggett
    Behind the Label

    Includes index
    ISBN 1 86381 003X

    1. Food — Composition. 2. Brand name products
    I. Leggett, Susan. II. Title

641.1

Typeset by Southern Media Services, Sydney
Schwartz Books is an imprint of
Southern Media Corporation Pty Ltd.

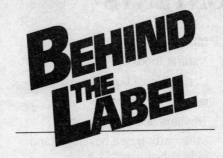

BEHIND THE LABEL

DR MARK LEGGETT
with SUSAN LEGGETT

SCHWARTZ BOOKS

CONTENTS

1.   Introduction 1
2.   Natural foods 5
3.   Conventional home prepared or
    manufactured foods 10
4.   Towards healtheir eating 17
5.   Milk, milk-based beverages and
    milk substitutes 22
6.   Breakfast cereals 31
7.   Breads, biscuits and cakes 65
8.   Spreads 78
9.   Cheeses 89
10. Crisps and savoury snacks 101
11. Soups 104
12. Main courses, convenience meals and
    packaged main course ingredients . . 117
13. Sauces, stocks and dressings 142
14. Desserts 155
15. Beverages 165
16. Confectionery 169
17. Approved products 176
    References 184
    Appendix I 185

1

Introduction

Information linking intakes of certain food factors with disease comes to attention almost daily. We now all know, for example, that excess fat intakes are linked to heart and circulatory system disease and that excess sugar consumption contributes to obesity.

But even when we are convinced, that knowledge is in fact useless without two other sorts of information:

- what is excess consumption

- how can we tell if we're exceeding the limits

And even where nutritional labelling is given on the packaging of the food we buy, this key information is still not provided. The purpose of this book is to provide this information.

In a previous book The Australian Food Report[1] we used the world's most definitive nutritional research results to identify the key food risk factors and their safe levels of consumption. For people in general, there really are only three key risks — fat, salt and excess energy intake. (Excess energy intake is largely caused by excess intake of fat, exacerbated by excess sugar.) For a quite small subset of people certain food additives such as some colourings and flavourings are also risk factors (these additives are listed in Appendix I).

Fat is implicated in heart and circulatory system disease and in some cancers. Salt (sodium) is implicated in high blood pressure. Excess kilojoule (energy) intake is implicated in obesity and linked to further factors causing shorter life expectancies. These three factors together are responsible for the vast majority of diet-related disease and death. They are also widespread (and in too high concentrations) across significant sections of the entire Australian food supply.

The guidelines from definitive world research used to assess foods in this book are outlined in the following table. The key risk factors fat, sodium and energy are covered. Cholesterol and sugars risk levels are given. Fibre levels are considered to assess which foods are significant sources. Finally, where additives are present, any potential health risks are clearly highlighted.

Table 1: Levels of intake of key food factors, existing and recommended

Diet type	Example	Energy kj/100g	Fat g/100g	Cholesterol g/100g	Sodium g/100g	Sugars g/100g	Fibre g/100g
Baseline	Present Australian diet[1]	713	7.0	.044	.250	8.1	1.28
Typical Moderate diet	Australian Department Health Target 2000[1]	Not stated	6.1	N.S..	.120	7.0	2.25
Levels Humans adapted to	Hunter-gatherer diet[2]	Not known	3.2	.045	.030	3.1	3.45
Earlier optimum diet plan	Pritikin diet[3]	300+	<2.0	.001	.090	4.4	Not stated
1990 optimum diet plan	Lifestyle Heart Trial[4]	No restriction	1.6	.001	.120	5.5	Not stated
Consensus energy optimum	eg. Doll and Peto[5]	600					
Consensus cholesterol target	eg. Briggs and Wahlqvist[6]			.015			
Soluble fibre target	eg. Anderson and others[7]						50g/day
The best practice dietary guidelines used in this book		600	2.0	.015	.120	5.0(sav.) 11.40 (sweet)	3.75g/100g* (Total)

* Level indicates a relatively high fibre food

Armed with these easily read guidelines we may now turn to the foods, both natural (unprocessed) and manufactured, that make up the Australian diet.

In the chapters that follow, we review a wide-ranging and representative cross-section of foods significant in the Australian food supply, indicating which are within the risk-factor guidelines and which are not. This review can be used to check the individual foods in your larder, and those you may consider buying. We conclude the review with a 'shopping list' of within guideline foods. Use of the list enables the selection of a wide range of healthy manufactured food products with confidence that you are not inadvertently exceeding health guidelines because of hidden health risk factors in the foods you buy.

2

Natural foods

A survey of published food analysis tables (e.g.[9]) shows that most fresh fruits and vegetables are within or near the guidelines used in this book and so in general may be used freely in the diet.

The same is not true, for at least some food factors, for meats, for eggs, and for nuts, and so these should be used only in strict moderation. The following examples for each food type illustrate these points, and provide more specific advice on usage.

Lean Deli Beef

Advertising claim: "95% fat free, 20% less salt"

Food Factor	Energy	Fat	Cholest.	Sodium	Sugars	Fibre
Labelling	435	4.0	N.S. (.059)	1.030	<1	N.S. (0)
Guideline	600	2.0	.015	.120	5.0	3.75
Conclusion	*	[ ]	[ ]	[ ]	*	N.A.

Additive Code		450	318	250
Translation		Sodium polyphosphate	Sodium erythorbate	Sodium nitrite
Function		Stabiliser accel.	Colour fixing	Curing agent, pres.
Conclusion		see page x	*	see page x

*Several above-guideline food components, as well as
additives lacking generally recognised-as-safe status.
Not recommended.*

Typical fruit 1: Apple (eating)

Food Factor	Energy	Fat	Cholest.	Sodium	Sugar	Fibre	Addit.
Content	196	0	0	.002	11.8	2.0	None
Guideline	600	2.0	.015	.120	11.40	3.75	
Conclusion	*	*	*	*	=	N.A.	*

Sugars at dessert-food guideline level. All other food factors well within guidelines. Recommended.

Typical fruit 2: Cherry (eating)

Food Factor	Energy	Fat	Cholest.	Sodium	Sugar	Fibre	Addit.
Content	201	0	0	.003	11.9	1.7	None
Guideline	600	2.0	.015	.120	11.40	3.75	
Conclusion	*	*	*	*	=	N.A.	*

Sugars at dessert-food guideline level. All other food factors well within guidelines. Recommended.

Typical leaf vegetable: Cabbage (savoy)

Food Factor	Energy	Fat	Cholest.	Sodium	Sugar	Fibre	Addit.
Content	109	0	0	.023	3.3	3.1	None
Guideline	600	2.0	.015	.120	5.0	3.75	
Conclusion	*	*	*	*	*	*	*

All food factors within guidelines. Use freely.

Typical root vegetable: Carrot

Food Factor	Energy	Fat	Cholest.	Sodium	Sugar	Fibre	Addit.
Content	98	0	0	.095	5.4	2.9	None
Guideline	600	2.0	.015	.120	5.0	3.75	
Conclusion	*	*	*	*	=	N.A.	*

Food factors either near or well within guidelines. Use freely.

Typical starchy vegetable: Potato
(boiled no added salt)

Food Factor	Energy	Fat	Cholest.	Sodium	Sugar	Fibre	Addit.
Content	438	0.4	0	.013	0.4	1.0	None
Guideline	600	2.0	.015	.120	5.0	3.75	
Conclusion	*	*	*	*	*	N.A.	*

Food factors within guidelines. Use freely.

Typical wild meat: Rabbit

Food Factor	Energy	Fat	Cholest.	Sodium	Sugar	Fibre	Addit.
Content	520	4.0	.071	.067	0	0	None
Guideline	600	2.0	.015	.120	5.0	3.75	
Conclusion	*	[]	[]	*	*	N.A.	*

Elevated in fat and cholesterol. Among the lowest of meats in these factors, hence recommended for use only as not- more than one-fifth of otherwise zero fat and cholesterol dish.

Typical low-fat fish: Cod
(baked without added fat)

Food Factor	Energy	Fat	Cholest.	Sodium	Sugar	Fibre	Addit.
Content	408	1.2	.060	.080	0	0	None
Guideline	600	2.0	.015	.120	5.0	3.75	
Conclusion	*	*	[]	*	*	N.A.	*

Except for cholesterol, within guidelines. Because few or no fish are lower in cholesterol, recommended as not more than one-quarter of otherwise zero cholesterol dish.

Typical domestic meat: Rump steak (grilled including fat)

Food Factor	Energy	Fat	Cholest.	Sodium	Sugar	Fibre	Addit.
Content	912	12.1	.082	.055	0	0	None
Guideline	600	2.0	.015	.120	5.0	3.75	
Conclusion	[]	[]	[]	*	*	N.A.	*

Elevated in several food factors, most notably in fat. As lower-fat meats exist, not recommended.

Egg, boiled

Food Factor	Energy	Fat	Cholest.	Sodium	Sugar	Fibre	Addit.
Content	612	10.9	.450	.140	0	0	None
Guideline	600	2.0	.015	.120	5.0	3.75	
Conclusion	=	[]	[]	=	*	N.A.	*

Elevated in fat and, famously, cholesterol (30 times the guide-line). As lower fat and cholesterol eggs do not yet exist, recommended for use but only at rate of one per week in otherwise within-guideline diet.

Typical nut: Peanuts, fresh

Food Factor	Energy	Fat	Cholest.	Sodium	Sugar	Fibre	Addit.
Content	2364	49.0	0	.006	3.1	8.1	None
Guideline	600	2.0	.015	.120	5.0	3.75	
Conclusion	[]	[]	*	*	*	*	*

Markedly elevated in energy and fat. For special occasions only.

3

Conventional home-prepared or manufactured foods

The point was illustrated in Chapter 2 that many fresh, unprocessed foods — primarily plant foods — are within the guidelines used in this book. The exact reverse is true of most conventional foods, whether manufactured or prepared at home. Most food types are significantly above at least one guideline, and many are simultaneously above several. The following brief survey illustrates these points. A detailed survey is available elsewhere (*The Australian Food Report* [1]).

In the present survey, we discuss an average example of each major category of manufactured food. These are: breakfast cereals; jams; milks; breads; biscuits and cakes; cheeses; crisps and savoury snacks; soups; main meals; desserts; beverages; and confectionery.

Typical breakfast cereal: cornflakes

Food Factor	Energy	Fat	Cholest.	Sodium	Sugar	Fibre	Addit.
Content as							
consumed*	448	.26	.001	.250	8.27	.63	None
Guideline	600	2.0	.015	.120	11.40	3.75	
Conclusion	*	*	*	[ ]	*	N.A.	*

* with skim milk and sugar

Cornflakes illustrates the key point that most conventional breakfast cereals are above guideline in sodium and hence, not recommended.

Conventional jam: Blackberry

Food Factor	Energy	Fat	Cholest.	Sodium	Sugar	Fibre	Addit.
Content							
on bread	940	1.78	0	.0017	10.6	7.7	None
Guideline	600	2.0	.015	.120	11.40	3.75	
Conclusion	[ ]	*	*	*	*	*	*

Except for energy, and this contributed mostly from bread, a straight-within guideline profile. For use in moderation, recommended.

Conventional whole milk

Food Factor	Energy	Fat	Cholest.	Sodium	Sugar	Fibre	Addit.
Content	281	3.8	.014	.056	4.6	0	None
Guideline	600	2.0	.015	.120	11.40	3.75	
Conclusion	*	[ ]	*	*	*	*	*

Elevated fat. As low fat milk is readily available, not recommended.

Conventional bread: white

Food Factor	Energy	Fat	Cholest.	Sodium	Sugar	Fibre	Addit.
Content	1017	1.5	.015	.507	1.8	2.7	various
Guideline	600	2.0	.015	.120	5.0	3.75	
Conclusion	[ ]	*	*	[ ]	*	N.A.	*

Elevated in energy and, fundamentally, in sodium due to added salt. Not recommended.

Conventional bread: wholemeal

Food Factor	Energy	Fat	Cholest.	Sodium	Sugar	Fibre	Addit.
Content	918	2.7	.015	.540	2.1	8.5	various
Guideline	600	2.0	015	.120	5.0	3.75	
Conclusion	[ ]	[ ]	*	[ ]	*	*	*

Elevated in fat and energy due to intrinsic qualities of wheat. But as for white bread, avoidably elevated in sodium due to added salt. Not recommended.

Conventional biscuit: gingernut

Food Factor	Energy	Fat	Cholest.	Sodium	Sugar	Fibre	Addit.
Content	1923	15.2	Not known	.330	36.8	2.0	various
Guideline	600	2.0	.015	.120	11.40	3.75	
Conclusion	[ ]	[ ]	[ ]	[ ]	[ ]	N.A.	*

Most food factors markedly elevated. Not recommended.

Typical cake: plain fruit cake

Food Factor	Energy	Fat	Cholest.	Sodium	Sugar	Fibre	Addit.
Content	1490	12.9	Not known	.250	43.1	2.8	various
Guideline	600	2.0	.015	.120	11.40	3.75	
Conclusion	[]	[]	[] probably	[]	[]	N.A.	*

Markedly elevated in all food factors. Not recommended.

Typical cheese: cheddar

Food Factor	Energy	Fat	Cholest.	Sodium	Sugar	Fibre	Addit.
Content	1682	33.5	.070	.610	Trace	0	None
Guideline	600	2.0	.015	.120	5.0	3.75	
Conclusion	[]	[]	[]	[]	*	N.A.	*

Most food factors above guidelines. Not recommended.

Typical savoury snack: potato crisps

Food Factor	Energy	Fat	Cholest.	Sodium	Sugar	Fibre	Addit.
Content	2224	35.9	Not known	.550	.7	11.9	None
Guideline	600	2.0	.015	.120	5.0	3.75	
Conclusion	[]	[]	[] probably	[]	*	*	*

Massively elevated energy, fat and sodium. Not recommended.

Typical soup: Cream of chicken

Food Factor	Energy	Fat	Cholest.	Sodium	Sugar	Fibre	Addit.
Content	242	3.8	Not known	.410	.7	0	various
Guideline	600	2.0	.015	.120	5.0.	3.75	
Conclusion	*	[ ]	* probably	[ ]	*	N.A.	*

Elevated fat and, principally, sodium. Not recommended.

Typical main course: Roast chicken and vegetables

Food Factor	Energy	Fat	Cholest.	Sodium	Sugar	Fibre	Addit.
Content	700	9.2	.030	.205	1.11	2.0	None
Guideline	600	2.0	.015	.120	5.0	3.75	
Conclusion	[ ]	[ ]	[ ]	[ ]	*	N.A.	*

Elevated in several food factors. Not recommended.

Conventional yeast extract: Marmite

Food Factor	Energy	Fat	Cholest.	Sodium	Sugar	Fibre	Addit.
Content	837	.5	0	4.400	5.2	—	None
As consumed*	909	1.83	0	.504	3.51	7.6	
Guideline	600	2.0	.015	.120	5.00	3.75	
Conclusion	[ ]	*	*	[ ]	*	*	*

* on salt-free bread (no butter)

Elevated in energy (because bread itself is). But even after dilution to a tenth, the sodium level of bread and Marmite is still markedly above guidelines. Not recommended.

Typical beverage I: packaged orange juice (no added sugar)

Food Factor	Energy	Fat	Cholest.	Sodium	Sugar	Fibre	Addit.
Content	184	0.3	0	.002	10.9	0	None
Guideline	600	2.0	.015	.120	11.40	3.75	
Conclusion	*	*	*	*	*	N.A.	*

Within all guidelines. Recommended.

Typical beverage II: standard cordial

Food Factor	Energy	Fat	Cholest.	Sodium	Sugar	Fibre
Content	117	0	0	<.010	7.2	0
Guideline	600	2.0	.015	.120	11.40	3.75
Conclusion	*	*	*	*	*	N.A.

Additive Code	330	211	223
Translation	Citric acid	Sodium benzoate	Sodium metabisulphite
Function	Flavour	Preservative	Preservative
Conclusion	see Appendix I	see Appendix I	see Appendix I

Additive Code	122	102	133
Translation	Azorubine	Tartrazine	Azo dye
Function	Colour	Colour	Colour
Conclusion	see Appendix I	see Appendix I	see Appendix I

Within guidelines for all food factors except additives.

Typical confectionery I: Milk chocolate

Food Factor	Energy	Fat	Cholest.	Sodium	Sugar	Fibre	Addit.
Content	2214	30.3	.140	.120	56.5	0	various
Guideline	600	2.0	.015	.120	11.40	3.75	
Conclusion	[ ]	[ ]	[ ]	=	[ ]	N.A.	*

Numerous above-guideline food factors. Not recommended,
except for very special occasions.

Typical confectionery II: Pastilles

Food Factor	Energy	Fat	Cholest.	Sodium	Sugar	Fibre	Addit.
Content	1079	0	0	.077	61.9	0	None
Guideline	600	2.0	.015	.120	11.40	3.75	
Conclusion	[ ]	*	*	*	[ ]	N.A.	*

Fewer above-guideline food factors than, say, chocolate.
Sugar and energy elevated, however. Not recommended
except for special occasions.

4

Towards healthier eating

Of the entire range of natural foods taken as they come, Chapter 2 showed that only the following types generally fall within our guidelines for foods with minimum risk factors: fresh fruits; fresh vegetables; and, used only in moderation, wild meats and fish.

Chapter 3 illustrated the following points concerning conventional home-prepared and manufactured foods. As expected, many sweet foods are above guidelines in energy and sugars: but even more are above the fat guideline and some are above the sodium guideline. And, most savoury foods are above the fat and sodium guidelines.

This state of affairs has led to two main developments: the creation of modified recipes to enable healthier home cooking, and the increasing availability of food products claiming to be healthier.

The home-cooking recipe modifications (eg[1,2]) are simple and few (even if far-reaching):

- Limit fat intake by: removing all visible fat from meat and chicken (skin chicken as well) before cooking; grilling and dry-baking rather than roasting; using low-fat yoghurt instead of sour cream; and using little or no butter, margarine or other cooking fats or oils. Removing fat leads to grilled rump steak decreasing from 12,.1g/100g fat to 6.0; and roast chicken decreasing from 14.0g/100g fat to 4.0g/100g (light meat). These fat levels, while still above the guideline, are really as low as meats can go. Hence they are recommended for use at about one-fifth the proportion of an otherwise zero-fat, zero-cholesterol dish.

- Use no-fat, low-sodium sauces, gravies and mayonnaises, and low-fat, low-salt cheeses.

- Meat portions should be reduced by one-third to one-half and vegetable portions increased to compensate.

- Salt should not be added to cooking, or at the table, and sugar use should be kept within guidelines.

The following tables show the marked changes which a steak dish can undergo when following these guidelines.

Conventional steak, coleslaw salad and chips

Food Factor	Energy	Fat	Cholest.	Sodium	Sugar	Fibre	Addit.
Content	696	10.0	.038	.161	2.4	2.0	None
Guideline	600	2.0	.015	.120	5.0	3.75	
Conclusion	*	[]	[]	[]	*	N.A.	*

Prudent-diet-style lean steak, coleslaw salad (no oil) and fat-free (grilled) chips

Food Factor	Energy	Fat	Cholest.	Sodium	Sugar	Fibre	Addit.
Content	312	1.23	.017	.041	2.6	2.27	None
Guideline	600	2.0	.015	.120	5.0	3.75	
Conclusion	*	*	*	*	*	N.A.	*

Concerning manufactured foods, the recommendation is again simple. No food should be in your larder unless it has been thoroughly vetted for the presence of the key relevant health-risk factors — and has passed the test *for each factor*.

Such a survey forms the purpose of the remainder of this book.

In conducting the survey the following approach was used.

Our 1989 laboratory test survey[1] of the labelling accuracy of Australian manufactured foods utilised over 100 specially commissioned analyses. This substantial survey showed that most (86 per cent) of claimed nutritional information (on levels of fat, sodium and sugars) was accurate (actual levels at, or not more than, levels stated on packaging).

Based on this survey result, our assessment policy for the present survey of manufactured foods was as follows.

1.   Foods were generally selected for review only if they contained a numerical nutritional labelling panel. (A manufactured food without it, whatever the advertising claim, should not be considered for inclusion in the larder.) We also reviewed some foods without nutritional labelling if they claimed improvements over conventional types (e.g. yeast extracts claiming reduced salt).

2.   Given the results of the 1989 laboratory test survey, which showed 86 per cent of labelling was accurate concerning the levels of food factors claimed, in this survey, levels on nutritional labelling were generally taken as read. The rationale of the present survey was to compare all claimed relevant food factor levels with our guidelines (see Chapter 1). Only those foods passing the guidelines for *each* risk factor are recommended for use.

3.   For a small number of new food types of potential special significance in the diet, a contract independent laboratory was engaged to carry out analytical tests on selected food omponents to check levels claimed on labelling.

4.   Fibre levels of foods are treated differently. For each food, it is simply noted whether or not the food is a good source of fibre. Foods

"lose no points" if they are not good sources of fibre as not all foods are expected to be.

5. Additives. No additives are deleterious for all people. Hence no additive is given a block ('not recommended') rating. Additives which may be deleterious *to some consumers* are given a 'see page X' reference where readers are given more information on the additive concerned to aid their own decision.

In each chapter which follows the key health risk associated with the food group in question is first discussed. Then a representative range of products in the group is reviewed, each food being given a star rating and either recommended or not recommended.

At the end of the book, all recommended foods are brought together in a shopping list format for your convenience.

For the survey, manufactured food products are reviewed in the following standard groupings: milk, milk-based beverages and milk substitutes; breakfast cereals; breads, biscuits and cakes; spreads; cheeses; crisps and savoury snacks; soups; main courses; convenience meals and packaged main-course ingredients; sauces, stocks and dressings; desserts; beverages; and confectionery.

5

Milks, milk-based beverages and milk substitutes

The main health risk-related issue with milk and milk products is the fat level, because milk fat contains a significant saturated proportion. For this reason, reduced fat and skimmed milk products have come onto the market in recent years. As well, entirely non-dairy milk substitutes have emerged.

The following survey reviews a substantial cross-section of these product types.

Betta Hi-Lo reduced Fat Modified Milk

Advertising claim: "70% less fat than regular milk"

Food Factor	Energy	Fat	Cholest.	Sodium	Sugar	Fibre	Addit.
Labelling	220	1.5	.006 (calc.)	.060	5.8	0	None
Guideline	600	2.0	.015	.120	5.0	3.75	
Conclusion	*	*	*	*	[]	N.A.	*

All food factors within guidelines except sugars. Not recommended.

Sanitarium So Good

Advertising claim: "No cholesterol. No lactose"

Food Factor	Energy	Fat	Cholest.	Sodium	Sugar	Fibre	Addit.
Labelling	260	3.4	0	.040	1.6	N.S.	None
Guideline	600	2.0	.015	.120	5.0	3.75	
Conclusion	*	[]	*	*	*	N.A.	*

Fat level above guideline. Not recommended.

Sanitarium So Good Lite Low Fat Soy Drink

Advertising claim: "Low fat; no cholesterol or lactose"

Food Factor	Energy	Fat	Cholest.	Sodium	Sugar	Fibre	Addit.
Labelling	180	0.7	0	.040	2	N.S.	None
Guideline	600	2.0	.015	.120	5*.0	3.75	
Conclusion	*	*	*	*	*	N.A.	*

Commendably, Sanitarium have produced a reduced fat version of standard So Good. An all-star profile. Recommended.

Bulla Thickened Lite Cream

Advertising claim: "48% less fat than regular thickened cream"

Food Factor	Energy	Fat	Cholest.	Sodium	Sugar	Fibre
Labelling	785	18.0	N.S. (.033)	.043	4.1	0
Guideline	600	2.0	.015	.120	5.0	3.75
Conclusion	[]	[]	[]	*	*	N.A.

Additive Code	441
Translation	Gelatine
Function	Thickener
Conclusion	*

Marked improvement in fat level over standard 35% fat cream. Recommended for use as ingredient (e.g. topping) at rate of 10 per cent or less of otherwise zero fat dish.

Red Seal Nutrisoy Non-dairy Instant Food Drink

Food Factor	Energy	Fat	Cholest.	Sodium	Sugar	Fibre	Addit.
Labelling	562	4.15	0	.019	17.6	N.S. (O)	None
Guideline	600	2.0	.015	.120	5.0	3.75	
Conclusion	*	[]	*	*	[]	N.A.	*

Above guideline fat and sugars. Not recommended.

Vitasoy Natural Soy Drink Creamy original

Advertising claim: "Cholesterol and lactose free"

Food Factor	Energy	Fat	Cholest.	Sodium	Sugar	Fibre	Addit.
Labelling	110	5	0	.115	10	*N.S.*	None
Guideline	600	2.0	.015	.120	11.40	3.75	
Conclusion	*	[]	*	*	*	N.A.	*

Elevated fat level. Not recommended.

Farmland Pasteurised Thickened Light Cream

Food Factor	Energy	Fat	Cholest.	Sodium	Sugar	Fibre
Labelling	785	18.0	.033	.043	4.1	0.
Guideline	600	2.0	.015	.120	5.0	3.75
Conclusion	[]	[]	[]	*	*	N.A.

Additive Code	441
Translation	Gelatine
Function	Thickener
Conclusion	*

*Significant fat reduction on that of normal whipping cream.
Recommended for use as no more than 10 per cent ingredient
of otherwise no-fat recipe.*

Tasmaid Form Reduced Fat Modified Milk

Food Factor	Energy	Fat	Cholest.	Sodium	Sugar	Fibre	Addit.
Labelling	205	1.2	*N.S.*	.062	5.4	0	None
Guideline	600	2.0	.015	.120	5.0	3.75	
Conclusion	*	*	*	*	[]	N.A.	*

*Energy, fat and sodium within guidelines, but sugar slightly
outside. Not recommended.*

Sanitarium So Good Flavoured Non-dairy Soy Drink — Honeycomb

Food Factor	Energy	Fat	Cholest.	Sodium	Sugar	Fibre
Labelling	300	3.2	0	.055	5.5	N.S.
Guideline	600	2.0	.015	.120	11.40	3.75
Conclusion	*	[ ]	*	*	*	N.A.

Additive Code	338	450	504	529
Translation	Phosphoric acid	Polyphosphate	Magnesium Carbonate	Calcium oxide
Function	Acidulent	Buffer	Anti-caking agent	Nutrient
Conclusion	*	*	*	*

Additive Code	509	102	110
Translation	Calcium chloride	Tartrazine	Sunset yellow
Function	Firming agent	Colour	Colour
Conclusion	*	see Appendix I	

see Appendix I

Elevated fat level. Not recommended.

Pure Harvest Traditional Pure Soy Vanilla Drink

Advertising claim: "Certified organic; no added sugar, no cholesterol or lactose."

Food Factor	Energy	Fat	Cholest.	Sodium	Sugar	Fibre	Addit.
Labelling	305	2.3	0	.074	10.0	N.S.	None
Guideline	600	2.0	.015	.120	11.40	3.75	
Conclusion	*	=	*	*	*	N.A.	*

No food components outside guidelines. Recommended.

Rev UHT Reduced Fat Calcium Enriched Modified Milk

Food Factor	Energy	Fat	Cholest.	Sodium	Sugar	Fibre	Addit.
Labelling	207	1.2	N.S. (.007)	.060	5.7	0	None
Guideline	600	2.0	.015	.120	5.0	3.75	
Conclusion	*	*	*	*	*	N.A.	*

Sugar above guideline. Not recommended.

Fit 4 Ultra Filtered Low Fat Milk

Advertising claim: "High protein, high calcium. only .9% fat."

Food Factor	Energy	Fat	Cholest.	Sodium	Sugar	Fibre	Addit.
Labelling	197	0.9	N.S. (<.015)	.043	4.7	*N.S.*	*None*
Guideline	600	2.0	.015	.120	5.0	3.75	
Conclusion	*	*	*	*	*	N.A.	*

A commendable within-guideline profile. Recommended.

Diploma Challenge SuperFiltered Milk

Food Factor	Energy	Fat	Cholest.	Sodium	Sugar	Fibre	Addit.
Labelling	243	1.2	N.S.(.007)	.080	6.9	0	None
Guideline	600	2.0	.015	.120	5.0	3.75	
Conclusion	*	*	*	*	[]	*	*

"Superfiltration" raises sodium and sugar levels above those of ordinary milk. Sodium remains within guidelines (as are energy and fat) but sugar is outside Guideline level for a plain milk. . Not recommended.

Berri Supreme Vanilla Non-dairy Soy Drink

Advertising claim: "No added salt, vegetable oil or cane sugar"

Food Factor	Energy	Fat	Cholest.	Sodium	Sugar	Fibre	Addit.
Labelling	300	0.2	0	.030	2.0	2.7	None
Guideline	600	2.0	.015	.120	11.4	3.75	
Conclusion	*	*	*	*	*	N.A.	*

Within guideline profile. Recommended. Note that unlike cow's milk, soy milks contain some fibre (from their bean origin remain) as a further benefit.

Westbrae Natural Lite All Natural Soy Drink (Plain)

Food Factor	Energy	Fat	Cholest.	Sodium	Sugar	Fibre	Addit.
Labelling	504	.40	0	.020	3.17	*N.S.*	None
Guideline	600	2.0	.015	.120	5.0	3.75	
Conclusion	*	*	*	*	*	N.A.	*

An all-within guideline profile. Recommended.

Suncoast Trim Reduced Fat Modified Milk

Food Factors	Energy	Fat	Cholest.	Sodium	Sugar	Fibre	Addit.
Labelling	220	1.6	N.S. (.008)	.052	4.8	N.S. (O)	None
Guideline	600	2.0	.015	.120	5.0	3.75	
Conclusion	*	*	*	*	*	N.A.	*

All within-guideline rating. Recommended.

Suncoast Shape High Calcium Low Fat Modified Milk

Food Factor	Energy	Fat	Cholest.	Sodium	Sugar	Fibre	Addit.
Labelling	195	0.15	N.S. (.002)	.052	4.8	N.S.	None (O)
Guideline	600	2.0	.015	.120	5.0	3.75	
Conclusion	*	*	*	*	*	N.A.	*

Six-star rating. Recommended.

Baco Reduced Fat Luxury Chocolate Flavoured Dairy Drink

Food Factor	Energy	Fat	Cholest.	Sodium	Sugar	Fibre
Labelling	227	1.9	*N.S.* (.008)	.055	9.3	N.S.(O)
Guideline	600	2.0	.015	.120	11.40	3.75
Conclusion	*	*	*	*	*	N.A.

Additive Code	471	407
Translation	Fatty acid glycerides	Irish moss
Function	Emulsifier	suspension agent
Conclusion	*	*

All-star profile. Recommended.

Pauls Go Lite Iced Coffee Flavoured Low Fat Modified Milk

Advertising claim: "Sweetened with Nutrasweet"

Food Factor	Energy	Fat	Cholest.	Sodium	Sugar	Fibre
Labelling	196	0.14	N.A. (.002)	.051	6.7	N.S.
Guideline	600	2.0	.015	.120	11.40	3.75
Conclusion	*	*	*	*	*	N.A.

Additive Code	407	
Translation	Irish moss	Aspartame
Function	Suspension agent	Sweetener
Conclusion	*	see Appendix I

Within guideline profile. Except for the minority for whom Aspartane is a problem, recommended.

Nippy's Iced Chocolate Flavoured Dairy Drink

Food Factor	Energy	Fat	Cholest.	Sodium	Sugar	Fibre	Addit.
Labelling	280	1.8	N.S. (<.015)	.056	9.8	N.S. (0)	Flavour
Guideline	600	2.0	.015	.120	11.4	3.75	
Conclusion	*	*	*	*	*	N.A.	*

Commendable six-star profile. Recommended.

6

Breakfast Cereals

Although by volume one's bowl of breakfast cereal
and milk appears to be mostly cereal with a little
milk in there somewhere, by weight the story is
different. A recommended serving of cereal is about
30g of cereal and half a cup (125g) of milk. By
weight then the cereal represents only 20 per cent of
the total. In a sense, your bowl of cereal is not a solid
food, but a crunchy milkshake.

All this is to say that because of this dilution by milk
the traditional characteristics of breakfast cereals are
more nearly those of milk than of the dry cereal
ingredients. For this reason, our assessments are
based on the nutritional profile of cereals as served.
The serving is with the recommended 125g of
(skimmed) milk, and, for plain cereals, with one
teaspoon of sugar.

As outlined in Chapter 3, the level of sodium is the
main issue with breakfast cereals. Added oat bran
has also been a recent marketing theme: for oat bran
products we estimate whether enough water-soluble
fibre has been provided to meet the daily target
researchers say is required[7].

A further point is that the cholesterol level is often not given on nutritional labelling. However cholesterol levels in cereal are rarely if ever significant. For this reason, it is our policy that a cereal will be recommended if it has an otherwise 'clean bill of health' even if the cholesterol level is not stated on the packaging.

Uncle Tobys Vitabrits

Advertising claim: "No added sugar"

Food Factor	Energy	Fat	Cholest.	Sodium	Sugar	Fibre	Addit.
Labelling	1370	1.4	N.S.	.450	1.5	10.0	None
As consumed with							
milk & sugar	421	.341	N.K.	.125	7.3	1.89	
Guideline	600	2.0	.015	.120	11.40	3.75	
Conclusion	*	*	N.K.	*	*	N.A.	*

Although close for sodium, Vitabrits, a long familiar breakfast classic, is within all guidelines. Recommended.

Kellogg's Rice Bubbles

Advertising claim: "Low in sugar; wholesome"

Food Factor	Energy	Fat	Cholest.	Sodium	Sugar	Fibre	Addit.
Labelling	1505	1.33	N.S.	1.092	9.99	3.33	None
As consumed with							
milk & sugar	452	0.325	N.K.	.246	8.91	.625	
Guideline	600	2.0	.015	.120	11.40	3.75	
Conclusion	*	*	N.K.	[ ]	*	*	*

Despite Kellogg's "wholesome" claim, because of the sodium level in Rice Bubbles, not recommended.

Kellogg's Just Right

Advertising claim: "Good source of fibre; low in fat"

Food Factor	Energy	Fat	Cholest.	Sodium	Sugar	Fibre	Addit.
Labelling	1509	2.3	0	.250	28.6	10.6	None
As consumed with							
milk only	408	.53	.001	.090	9.57	2.05	
Guideline	600	2.0	.015	.120	11.40	3.75	
Conclusion	*	*	*	*	*	N.A.	*

Consumed strictly without table-added sugar, Just Right falls within guidelines. Recommended.

Kellogg's Coco Pops

Food Factor	Energy	Fat	Cholest.	Sodium	Sugar	Fibre	Addit.
Labelling	1553	2.5	N.S.	.720	39	1.7	None
As consumed with							
milk	415	.129	N.K.	.181	11.58	.32	
Guideline	600	2.0	.015	.120	11.40	3.75	
Conclusion	*	*	N.K.	[ ]	=	N.A.	*

Because of the sodium level — not recommended.

Uncle Toby's Extra G

Advertising claim: "The low fat, high protein breakfast"

Food Factor	Energy	Fat	Cholest.	Sodium	Sugar	Fibre	Addit.
Labelling	1400	0.5	N.S.	.847	18.0	6.5	None
As consumed with
milk & sugar	426	.17	N.K.	.199	10.41	1.22	
Guideline	600	2.0	.015	.120	11.40	3.75	
Conclusion	*	*	N.K.	[ ]	*	N.A.	*

Low fat, high protein maybe, but also above guideline for sodium. Not recommended.

Kellogg's Froot Loops Fruit Flavoured Cereal

Food Factor	Energy	Fat	Cholest.	Sodium	Sugar	Fibre
Labelling	1625	4.33	0	.496	44.0	N.S.
As consumed with
milk only	430	.920	.001	.138	12.55	
Guideline	600	2.0	.015	.120	11.40	3.75
Conclusion	*	*	*	=	=	N.A.

Additive Code	110	102	127	133
Translation	Sunset Yellow	Tartrazine	Erythrosine	Brilliant Blue
Function	Colour	Colour	Colour	Colour
Conclusion	see Appendix I		see Appendix I	see Appendix I

As consumed, Froot Loops are within or near all guidelines. But the slew of additives may lead the prudent (even those non-allergic) to avoid.

Abundant Earth Puffed Wheat

Food Factor	Energy	Fat	Cholest.	Sodium	Sugar	Fibre	Addit.
Labelling	1500	2.2	N.S.	.0031	1.1	2.5	None
As consumed with							
milk & sugar	476	.54	N.K.	.041	7.26	.83	
Guideline	600	2.0	.015	.120	11.40	3.75	
Conclusion	*	*	N.K.	*	*	N.A.	*

All food factors within guidelines. Recommended.

Abundant Earth Puffed Millet

Food Factor	Energy	Fat	Cholest.	Sodium	Sugar	Fibre	Addit.
Labelling	1500	2.9	N.S.(O)	.010	1.1	3.2	None
As consumed with							
milk & sugar	476	.68	.001	.043	7.3	.67	
Guideline	600	2.0	.015	.120	11.40	3.75	
Conclusion	*	*	*	*	*	N.A.	*

Five star rating. Recommended.

Alevita Muesli with Fruit

	Energy	Fat	Cholest.	Sodium	Sugar	Fibre	Addit.
Labelling	1410	4.5	N.S.	.083	N.A.	N.A.	None
as consumed with							
milk only	751	1.95	N.K.	.076	N.A.	N.A.	
Guideline	600	2.0	.015	.120	11.40	3.75	
Conclusion	[ ]	*	N.K.	*	N.A.	N.A.	*

Elevated in energy. Not recommended.

Sanitarium Good Start Muesli Breakfast Biscuits

Food Factor	Energy	Fat	Cholest.	Sodium	Sugar	Fibre	Addit.
Labelling	1470	6.2	N.S	.350	9.4	9.9	None
As consumed with							
milk & sugar	602	2.0	N.K.	.145	8.89	3.13	
Guideline	600	2.0	.015	.120	11.40	.3.75	
Conclusion	=	=	N.K.	[ ]	*	=	*

A generally acceptable low-risk profile, but marred by the sodium level. On balance, not recommended.

Kellogg's All Bran

Food Factor	Energy	Fat	Cholest.	Sodium	Sugar	Fibre	Addit.
Labelling	1062	3.3	0	1.020	13.5	31.0	None
As consumed with							
milk & sugar	363	.696	.001	.232	9.56	5.82	
Guideline	600	2.0	.015	.120	11.40	3.75	
Conclusion	*	*	*	[ ]	*	*	*

A commendable source of fibre (which reduces disease risk) marred by a very high sodium level (which increases disease risk). Not recommended.

Farmland High Fibre Breakfast Bran with Sultanas

Food Factor	Energy	Fat	Cholest.	Sodium	Sugar	Fibre	Addit.
Labelling	1180	5.3	N.S.	.570	23.5	26.1	None
As consumed with							
milk only	343	1.72	N.K.	.142	13.30	5.0	
Guideline	600	2.0	.015	.120	11.40	3.75	
Conclusion	*	*	N.K.	[ ]	=	*	*

A generally well-balanced cereal, but marred by an above-guideline sodium level. For this reason, not recommended.

Uncle Toby's Fibre Plus

Advertising Claim: "High in fibre, low in fat"

Food Factor	Energy	Fat	Cholest.	Sodium	Sugar	Fibre	Addit.
Labelling	1320	5.3	N.S.	.250	24.0	17.7	None
As consumed with							
milk & sugar	411	.491	N.K.	.088	11.53	3.31	
Guideline	600	2.0	.015	.120	11.40	3.75	
Conclusion	*	*	N.K.	*	=	=	*

Despite being moderate rather than high in fibre as consumed, on overall profile Uncle Toby's Fibre Plus is recommended.

Uncle Toby's Multi Bran

Advertising claim: "No added salt, high in dietary fibre, cholesterol free"

Food Factor	Energy	Fat	Cholest.	Sodium	Sugar	Fibre (sol)	Addit.
Labelling	1480	12.2	Nil	.007	2.6	23.6 (4.8)	None
As consumed with milk & sugar	504	2.4	.001	.042	7.52	4.43 (.9)	
Guideline	600	2.0	.015	.120	11.40	3.75 (1.8)	
Conclusion	*	[ ]	*	*	*	* [ ]	*

Slightly high in fat, and two helpings a day would be required to meet soluble fibre target. With these provisos, on balance recommended.

Kellogg's Balance Oat Bran Flakes

Food Factor	Energy	Fat	Cholest.	Sodium	Sugars	Fibre (sol)	Addit.
Labelling	1596	3.3	0	.120	11.7	12.2 (6.4)	None
As consumed with milk & sugar	463	.703	.001	.063	9.23	1.20 (0.6)	
Guideline	600	2.0	.015	.120	11.40	3.75 (1.8)	
Conclusion	*	*	*	*	*	[ ][ ]	*

Except for fibre, a commendable low-risk profile. Recommended. However, three serves per day would be required to meet the soluble fibre target, and this is not made clear on the packaging.

Sanitarium Bran Cereal

Food Factor	Energy	Fat	Cholest.	Sodium	Sugar	Fibre
Labelling	1190	8.5	N.S.	.820	15.4	28.0
As consumed with						
milk & sugar	387	1.67	N.K.	194	9.9	5.25
Guideline	600	2.0	.015	.120	11.40	3.75
Conclusion	*	*	N.K.	[ ]	*	*

Additive Code	170
Translation	Calcium carbonate (colouring)
Conclusion	*

A commendable low-risk profile, except for sodium. And for this reason, not recommended.

Kellogg's Ready Wheats

Food Factor	Energy	Fat	Cholest	Sodium	Sugar	Fibre	Addit.
Labelling	1523	2.6	N.S.	.003	.9	9.3	None
As consumed with							
milk & sugar	449	.25	N.K.	.041	7.20	1.74	
Guideline	600	2.0	.015	.120	11.40	3.75	
Conclusion	*	*	N.K.	*	*	[ ]	*

An exemplary low-risk profile. Recommended.

Sanitarium Puffed Wheat,

Advertising claim: "No added salt, colourings, flavourings, sugar"

Food Factor	Energy	Fat	Cholest.	Sodium	Sugar	Fibre	Addit.
Labelling	1440	2.6	N.S.	.017	1.0	N.S.	None
As consumed with							
milk & sugar	434	.56	N.K.	.044	7.22		
Guideline	600	2.0	.015	.120	11.40	3.75	
Conclusion	*	*	N.K.	*	*	N.A.	*

A clear low-risk profile. Recommended.

Kellogg's Bran Flakes

Advertising claim: "Low in fat"

Food Factor	Energy	Fat	Cholest.	Sodium	Sugar	Fibre	Addit.
Labelling	1210	2.6	N.S.	.895	8.0	21.0	None
As consumed with							
milk & sugar	391	.566	N.K.	.208	8.53	3.94	
Guideline	600	2.0	.015	.120	11.40	3.75	
Conclusion	*	*	N.K.	[ ]	*	*	*

Because of sodium level, not recommended.

Sanitarium Light'n'Tasty Breakfast Cereal

Advertising claim: "10% oat bran"

Food Factor	Energy	Fat	Cholest.	Sodium	Sugar	Fibre
Labelling	1410	3.0	N.S.	.230	20.5.	.10.6
As consumed with						
milk & sugar	428	.64	N.K.	.084	10.88	1.99
Guideline	600	2.0	.015	.120	11.40	3.75
Conclusion	*	*	N.K.	*	*	N.A.

Additive Code	260	262
Translation	Acetic acid	Sodium diacetate
Function	Preservative	Preservative
Conclusion	*	*

Sanitarium Light'n'Tasty Breakfast Cereal has an excellent overall low-risk profile and is recommended. However, note that the 10 per cent oat bran is nowhere near enough, supplying only one-sixteenth of the daily requirement.

Kellogg's Honey Smacks

Advertising claim: "No preservatives. Contains vitamins and iron"

Food Factor	Energy	Fat	Cholest.	Sodium	Sugar	Fibre
Labelling	1611	4.66	N.S.	.033	52.9	1.67
As consumed with						
milk only	484	.98	N.K.	.048	14.3	.32
Guideline	600	2.0	.015	.120	11.40	3.75
Conclusion	*	*	N.K.	*	[ ]	N.A.

Additive Code	262		1400		
Translation	Sodium diacetate		Dextrin		Amino acid
Function	Preservative		Thickener		Texturiser
Conclusion	*		*		*

Known for its high sugar level as packaged, Kellogg's Honey Smacks sugar level as consumed is not markedly above guidelines thanks to the massive dilution effect of milk. And the cereal does have the virtue of a very low sodium level. A minor separate point is that 'no preservatives' is claimed. Yet additive 262 (while recognised as safe) is classed as a preservative in our references. Recommended.

Sanitarium Corn Flakes

Advertising claim: " . . . less salt than other corn flakes"

Food Factor	Energy	Fat	Cholest.	Sodium	Sugar	Fibre	Addit.
Labelling	1460	1.5	N.S.	.900	7.6	2.3	None
As consumed with							
milk & sugar	438	.359	N.K.	.209	9.14	.43	
Guideline	600	2.0	.015	.120	11.40	3.75	
Conclusion	*	*	N.K.	*	*	N.A.	*

*Sanitarium Corn Flakes may well have less salt than (some)
other cornflakes, but the slogan is surely unhelpful as the
sodium level is still well above the guideline. Not
recommended.*

Sanitarium Granose

Advertising claim: Absolutely no added sugar"

Food Factor	Energy	Fat	Cholest.	Sodium	Sugar	Fibre	Addit.
Labelling	1340	2.7	N.S.	.350	1.2	N.S.	None
As consumed with							
milk & sugar	415	.584	N.K.	.106	7.26		
Guideline	600	2.0	.015	.120	11.40	3.75	
Conclusion	*	*	N.K.	*	*	N.A.	*

A commendable low-risk profile. Recommended.

Kellogg's Corn Flakes

Advertising claim: "Kellogg's Corn Flakes are low in sugar and fat (two things nutritionists recommend we cut down on)"

Food Factors	Energy	Fat	Cholest.	Sodium	Sugar	Fibre	Addit.
Labelling	1516	1.3	0	1.133	6.6	3.3	None
As consumed with							
milk & sugar	448	.259	.001	.250	8.27	.63	
Guideline	600	2.0	.015	.120	11.40	3.75	
Conclusion	*	*	*	[ ]	*	N.A.	*

Kellogg's health message trumpets Corn Flakes' low fat and sugar levels, but is silent on the third of the trio, sodium. And even as consumed heavily dilutedwith milk, the sodium level is still over twice the guideline. Not recommended.

Uncle Toby's Vitabrits

Advertising claim: "No added sugar"

Food Factor	Energy	Fat	Cholest.	Sodium	Sugar	Fibre	Addit.
Labelling	1370	1.4	N.S.	.450	1.5	10.0	None
As consumed with							
milk & sugar	421	.341	N.K.	.120	7.3	1.89	
Guideline	600	2.0	.015	.120	11.40	3.75	
Conclusion	*	*	N.K.	*	*	N.A.	*

No food factor above guidelines. Recommended.

Kellogg's Frosties

Advertising claim: "Same sugar as an apple"

Food Factor	Energy	Fat	Cholest.	Sodium	Sugar	Fibre	Addit.
Labelling	1528	1.67	N.S.	.809	35.0	3.33	None
As consumed with							
milk only	411	.403	N.K.	.199	10.48	.650	
Guideline	600	2.0	.015	.120	11.40	3.75	
Conclusion	*	*	N.K.	[ ]	*	N.A.	*

Despite the consumer group focus on the added sugar of foods like Frosties, as consumed it is the sodium, not the sugar, which is above the guideline. Not recommended.

Sanitarium Weetbix

Food Factor	Energy	Fat	Cholest.	Sodium	Sugar	Fibre	Addit.
Labelling	1380	2.7	N.S.	.270	2.3	N.S.	None
As consumed with							
milk & sugar	423	.059	N.K.	.091	7.46		
Guideline	600	2.0	.015	.120	11.40	3.75	
Conclusion	*	*	N.K.	*	*	N.A.	*

The classic breakfast cereal effectively gets an all-star low-risk rating. Recommended.

Kellogg's Sustain

Advertising claim: "Keeps the energy in your day longer"

Food Factor	Energy	Fat	Cholest.	Sodium	Sugar	Fibre
Labelling	1461	4.3	0	.110	15.0	7.0
As consumed with						
milk & sugar	438	.89	.001	.061	9.3	1.44
Guideline	600	2.0	.015	.120	11.40	3.75
Conclusion	*	*	*	*	*	N.A.

Additive Code	469
Translation	Sodium caseinate
Function	Emulsifier
Conclusion	*

Kelloggs are really to be commended for this attractive low-risk cornflake alternative. Recommended.

Uncle Toby's Weeties

Advertising claim: "Each flake is one whole wheat grain with no added sugar"

Food Factor	Energy	Fat	Cholest.	Sodium	Sugar	Fibre	Addit.
Labelling	1386	1.67	N.S.	.513	3.0	N.S.	None
As consumed with							
milk I & sugar	416	0.5	N.K.	.154	0.9		
Guideline	600	2.0	.015	.120	11.40	3.75	
Conclusion	*	*	N.K.	[ ]	*	N.A.	*

Elevated sodium. Not recommended.

Kellogg's Puffed Wheat

Advertising claim: "No added sugar, salt, colourings,
flavourings, preservatives, or cholesterol"

Food Factor	Energy	Fat	Cholest.	Sodium	Sugar	Fibre	Addit.
Labelling	1614	2.3	0	.003	1.1	6.0	None
As consumed with							
milk & sugar	466	.510	.001	.041	7.24	1.12	
Guideline	600	2.0	.015	.120	11.40	3.75	
Conclusion	*	*	*	*	*		*

About as low-risk a breakfast as you can get. Highly
recommended.

Kellogg's Nutri Grain High Nutrition Cereal

Advertising claim: "High in protein"

Food Factor	Energy	Fat	Cholest.	Sodium	Sugar	Fibre
Labelling	1601	2.7	0	.666	35.0	N.S.
As consumed with						
milk & sugar	464	.58	.001	.165	21.8	
Guideline	600	2.0	.015	.120	11.40	3.75
Conclusion	*	*	*	[ ]	[ ]	N.A.

Additive Code	100	
Translation	Turmeric	Paprika
Function	Colour	Colour
Conclusion	*	*

While the high protein claim may be relevant to iron men,
even they don't need the sodium and sugar levels of Nutri
Grain. Not recommended.

Sanitarium Weetbix plus Oatbran

Food Factor	Energy	Fat	Cholest.	Sodium	Sugar	Fibre	Addit.
Labelling	1340	3.1	N.S.	.270	6.0	13.3	None
As consumed with							
milk & sugar	415	.663	N.K.	.091	8.16	2.5	
Guideline	600	2.0	.015	.120	11.40	3.75	
Conclusion	*	*	N.K.	*	*	N.A.	*

An admirable low-risk profile, and recommended. But note that as consumed, even oat-bran fortified Weetbix does not really provide the amount of fibre its title might suggest.

Kellogg's Special K

Advertising claim: "Low in fat"

Food Factor	Energy	Fat	Cholest.	Sodium	Sugar	Fibre	Addit.
Labelling	1597	2.0	N.S.	.750	14.0	1.6	None
As consumed with							
milk & sugar	494	.045	N.K.	.181	9.66	.3	
Guideline	600	2.0	.015	.120	11.40	3.75	
Conclusion	*	*	N.K.	[]	*	N.A.	*

Low in fat indeed, but not especially so for a cereal. And in the health atmosphere set up by the 'low' message, what about the sodium level? Not recommended.

Kellogg's Crunchy Nut Cornflakes

Food Factor	Energy	Fat	Cholest.	Sodium	Sugar	Fibre	Addit.
Labelling	1664	6.8	N.S.	.748	21.8	3.3	None
As consumed with							
milk & sugar	476	1.35	N.K.	.181	11.13	.63	
Guideline	600	2.0	.015	.120	11.40	3.75	
Conclusion	*	*	N.K.	[ ]	*	N.A.	*

Elevated sodium. Not recommended.

Sanitarium Weetbix Hi-bran

Food Factor	Energy	Fat	Cholest.	Sodium	Sugar	Fibre	Addit.
Labelling	1395	9.4	N.S.	.460	9.3	18.1	None
As consumed with							
milk &. sugar	426	1.84	N.K.	.127	8.78	3.39	
Guideline	600	2.0	.015	.120	11.40	3.75	
Conclusion	*	*	N.K.	=	*	N.A.	*

A generally low-risk profile, but those rigorously avoiding sodium may wish to choose other lower-sodium versions.

Sanitarium Lite Bix

Advertising claim: "Salt, sugar and fat among the lowest of any breakfast cereal"

Food Factor	Energy	Fat	Cholest.	Sodium	Sugar	Fibre	Addit.
Labelling	1340	2.7	N.S.	.020	1.2	12.0	None
As consumed with							
milk & sugar	415	.584	N.K.	.044	7.26	2.25	
Guideline	600	2.0	.015	.120	11.40	3.75	
Conclusion	*	*	N.K.	*	*	N.A.	*

A truly exemplary health breakfast cereal.
Highly recommended.

Uncle Toby's Rice Bran

Advertising claim: "Can help reduce cholesterol"

Food Factor	Energy	Fat	Cholest.	Sodium	Sugar	Fibre	Addit.
Labelling	1800	20.4	Nil	.008	4.0	25.5	None
As consumed with							
milk & sugar	320	3.4	.001	.010	3.36	4.25	
Guideline	600	2.0	.015	.120	11.40	3.75	
Conclusion	*	[ ]	*	*	*	*	*

Despite the genuinely high fibre level, above guideline fat. Not recommended.

Uncle Toby's Crunchy Oat Bran Cereal with Fruit

Advertising claim: "Can help reduce cholesterol"

Food Factor	Energy	Fat	Cholest.	Sodium	Sugar	Fibre (sol)	Addit.
Labelling	1520	6.0	N.S.	.352	22.0	12.5 (5.8)	None
As consumed with							
milk only	507	1.66	N.K.	.131	9.5	3.31 (1.54)	
Guideline	600	2.0	.015	.120	11.40	3.75 (1.8)	
Conclusion	*	*	N.K.	=	*	= =	*

No food component above guideline: recommended. Note that three serves daily would be needed to meet the soluble fibre guideline from Uncle Toby's Crunchy Oat Bran Cereal with Fruit alone.

Sun Farm Rice Bran

Advertising claim: "Gluten free"

Food Factor	Energy	Fat	Cholest.	Sodium	Sugar	Fibre	Addit.
Labelling	1774	20.4	0	.006	4.0	22.5	None
As consumed with							
milk & sugar	319	3.4	.001	.008	3.36	3.75	
Guideline	600	2.0	.015	.120	11.40	3.75	
Conclusion	*	[]	*	*	*	*	*

High fat content. Not recommended.

Uncle Toby's Oat Bran

Food Factor	Energy	Fat	Cholest.	Sodium	Sugar	Fibre (sol)	Addit.
Labelling	1480	8.6	0	.002	< 1	17.2 (9.2)	None
As consumed with							
milk & sugar	266	1.43	.001	.003	2.08	4.78 (2.6)	
Guideline	600	2.0	.015	.120	11.40	3.75 (1.8)	
Conclusion	*	*	*	*	*	**	*

An exemplary low-risk profile. And especially note that one recommended serve daily (involving 60g of dry oat bran in the recipe) would provide 5.5g of soluble fibre, above the target of 4.6g per day. Highly recommended.

Quaker Cream Oats

Advertising claim: 100% natural oats"

Food Factor	Energy	Fat	Cholest.	Sodium	Sugar	Fibre	Addit.
Labelling	1624	8.2	N.S.	.004	1.3	1.42	None
As consumed with							
milk & sugar	173	.76	N.K.	.028	2.88	.13	
Guideline	600	2.0	.015	.120	11.40	3.75	
Conclusion	*	*	N.K.	*	*	N.A.	*

A low-risk profile. Recommended.

Kellogg's Bran Flakes

Advertising claim: '"Low in fat"

Food Factor	Energy	Fat	Cholest.	Sodium	Sugar	Fibre	Addit.
Labelling	1210	2.6	N.S.	.895	8.0	21.0	None
As consumed with							
milk & sugar	391	.566	N.K.	.208	8.53	3.94	
Guideline	600	2.0	.015	.120	11.40	3.75	
Conclusion	*	*	N.K.	[]	*	*	*

Because of sodium level, not recommended.

Willow Valley Crunchy Toasted Oat Bran Breakfast Cereal

Food Factor	Energy	Fat	Cholest.	Sodium	Sugars	Fibre (sol)	Addit.
Labelling	1606	3.8	N.A.	.004	11.5	15.0 (7.5)	None
As consumed with milk & sugar	532	.99	N.K.	.036	8.88	3.65 (1.83)	
Guideline	600	2.0	.015	.120	11.40	3.75 (1.8)	
Conclusion	*	*	N.K.	*	*	* *	*

One of the best overall cereal profiles we have seen. Recommended. However, note that 2.5 serves daily would be needed to reach the soluble fibre target.

Willow Valley Crunchy Toasted Oat Bran Breakfast Cereal with Fruit

Food Factor	Energy	Fat	Cholest.	Sodium	Sugar	Fibre Total Sol.	Addit.
Labelling	1591	4.17	N.S.	.003	22.5	13.0 6.5	None
As consumed with milk only	526	1.18	.001	.039	9.63	3.44 1.72	
Guideline	600	2.0	.015	.120	11.40	3.75 1.8	
Conclusion	*	*	*	*	*	= =	*

A commendable overall profile, and recommended. Note, however, that 2.5 recommended serves a day would be needed to reach the soluble fibre target.

Kellogg's Balance Oat Bran Cereal with Fruit

Food Factor	Energy	Fat	Cholest.	Sodium	Sugar	Fibre	(Sol)
Labelling	1661	14.5	N.S.	.113	23.2	8.9	2.6
As consumed with							
milk & sugar	544	3.91	N.K.	.06	9.82	2.35	.7
Guideline	600	2.0	.015	.120	11.40	3.75	1.8
Conclusion	*	[ ]	N.K.	*	*	N.A.	N.A.

Additive Code	420
Translation	Sorbitol
Function	Humectant
Conclusion	see Appendix I

Elevated fat level. Not recommended. Note that six serves per day would be needed to reach the soluble fibre target from Balance with Fruit alone.

Purina Toasted Muesli Flakes

Food Factors	Energy	Fat	Cholest.	Sodium	Sugar	Fibre	Addit.
Labelling	1430	3.0	Nil	.338	28	8.0	None
As consumed with							
milk only	327	0.72	.001	.107	9.45	1.55	
Guideline	600	2.0	.015	.120	11.40	3.75	
Conclusion	*	*	*	*	*	N.A.	*

All risk factors within guidelines. Recommended.

Cerola Apricot Toasted Muesli

Advertising claim: "National Heart Foundation approved"

Food Factor	Energy	Fat	Cholest.	Sodium	Sugar	Fibre	Addit.
Labelling	1703	10.4	N.S.	.077	21.3	14.2	None
As consumed with							
milk only	648	3.44	N.K.	.040	10.29	4.67	
Guideline	600	2.0	.015	.120	11.40	3.75	
Conclusion	=	[ ]	N.K.	*	*	*	*

Above guideline fat level. Not recommended.

Cerola Natural Muesli

Advertising claim: "National Heart Foundation approved;
Good source of fibre"

Food Factor	Energy	Fat	Cholest.	Sodium	Sugar	Fibre	Addit.
Labelling	1590	8.7	N.S.	.161	21.4	10.6	None
As consumed with							
milk only	612	2.89	N.K.	.088	10.3	3.44	
Guideline	600	2.0	.015	.120	11.40	3.75	
Conclusion	*	[ ]	N.K.	*	*	=	*

Elevated fat level. Not recommended.

Kellogg's Komplete Muesli Country Style

Food Factor	Energy	Fat	Cholest.	Sodium	Sugar	Fibre
Labelling	1547	5.8	0	.019	24.7	9.4
As consumed with						
milk only	598	1.94	.001	.076	11.4	3.05
Guideline	600	2.0	.015	.120	11.40	3.75
Conclusion	=	=	*	*	=	=

Additive Code	322
Translation	Lecithin
Function	Antioxidant
Conclusion	*

For mueslis, which find it difficult to provide a balance between low enough fat and high enough fibre, this is a good overall profile. Recommended.

Purina Toasted Muesli

Advertising claim: "One-third less fat"

Food Factor	Energy	Fat	Cholest.	Sodium	Sugar	Fibre	Addit.
Labelling	1670	16.5	N.S.	.186	20.0	12.4	None
As consumed with							
milk only	638	5.42	N.K.	.096	9.86	4.02	
Guideline	600	2.0	.015	.120	11.40	3.75	
Conclusion	=	[ ]	N.K.	*	*	*	*

Purina Toasted Muesli may contain one-third less fat than other toasted mueslis, but this still does not bring its fat level within the guideline. Not recommended.

Willow Valley Crunchy Toasted Oat Bran Muesli

Advertising claim: "National Heart Foundation approved"
"High in soluble fibre; no added salt"

Food Factor	Energy	Pat	Cholest.	Sodium	Sugar	Fibre	Addit.
Labelling	1688	9.13	N.S.	.004	42.3.	13.0	None
As consumed with							
milk only	752	3.10	N.K.	.036	11.70	4.22	
Guideline	600	2.0	.015	.120	11.40	3.75	
Conclusion	[ ]	[ ]	N.K.	*	=	*	*

Elevated energy and fat. Despite National Heart Foundation approval, not recommended.

Cerola Toasted Muesli

Adver. ˸ing claim: "National Heart Foundation approved"

Food Factor	Energy	Fat	Cholest.	Sodium	Sugar	Fibre
Labelling	1700	9.3	N.S.	.097	20.4	13.4
As consumed with						
milk only	647	3.02	N.K.	.066	9.99	4.35
Guideline	600	2.0	.015	.120	11.40	3.75
Conclusion	=	[ ]	N.K.	*	*	*

Additive Code 322
Translation	Lecithin
Function	Antioxidant
Conclusion	*

Elevated fat level. Despite National Heart Foundation approval, not recommended.

Cerola Oat Bran Muesli

Advertising claim: "National Heart Foundation approved"

Food Factor	Energy	Fat	Cholest.	Sodium	Sugar	Fibre (sol)
Labelling	1641	9.4	N.S.	.066	18.3	13.4 (2.5)
As consumed with milk only	629	3.12	N.K.	.037	9.3	4.35 (.81)
Guideline	600	2.0	.015	.120	11.40	3.75 (1.8)
Conclusion	=	[ ]	N.K.	*	*	* [ ]

Additive Code 322
Translation   Lecithin
Function   Antioxidant
Conclusion   *

Elevated fat. Not recommended. Also note that three 60g helpings per day would be needed to reach the soluble fibre target.

Kellogg's Komplete Muesli (Oven Baked)

Food Factor	Energy	Fat	Cholest.	Sodium	Sugar	Fibre
Labelling	1931	21.0	0	.110	18	7.8
As consumed with						
milk only	722	6.88	.001	.071	17.05	2.53
Guideline	600	2.0	.015	.120	11.40	3.75
Conclusion	[ ]	[]	*	*	[ ]	N.A.

Additive Code	322	414	270
Translation	Lecithin	Gum arabic	Lactic acid
Function	Antioxidant	Stabiliser	Preservative
Conclusion	*	*	*

Elevated energy, fat and sugars, and lower-than-target fibre.
Not recommended.

Uncle Toby's Muesli Flakes

Food Factor	Energy	Fat	Cholest.	Sodium	Sugar	Fibre
Labelling	1390	2.6	N.S.	.240	19	9
As consumed with						
milk only	384	.58	N.K.	.088	7.71	1.74
Guideline	600	2.0	.015	.120	11.40	3.75
Conclusion	*	*	N.K.	*	*	N.A.

Additive Code	330
Translation	Sodium citrate
Function	Antioxidant
Conclusion	*

Commendable profile. Recommended.

Uncle Toby's Natural Muesli — True Swiss Formula

Food Factor	Energy	Fat	Cholest.	Sodium	Sugar	Fibre	Addit.
Labelling	1490	7.0	N.S.	.0337	21.3	10.7	None
As consumed with milk only	579	2.29	N.K.	.046	10.29	3.47	
Guideline	600	2.0	.015	.120	11.40	3.75	
Conclusion	*	=	N.K.	*	*	=	*

No risk factors significantly above guideline. Recommended.

Goodness Products Tropical Fruits Natural Muesli

Advertising claim: "No added salt, no added sugar; National Heart Foundation Approved"

Food Factor	Energy	Fat	Cholest.	Sodium	Sugar	Fibre	Addit.
Labelling	1477	8.1	N.S.	.011	18.5	8.5	None
As consumed with milk only	575	2.69	N.K.	.039	9.34	2.76	
Guideline	600	2.0	.015	.120	11.40	3.75	
Conclusion	*	[ ]	N.K.	*	*	N.A.	*

Elevated fat level. Not recommended.

Uncle Toby's Natural Muesli Apricot and Almond

Food Factor	Energy	Fat	Cholest.	Sodium	Sugar	Fibre	Addit.
Labelling	1470	8.0	N.S.	.0326	19.3	12.3	None
As consumed with							
milk only	573	2.66	N.K.	.046	9.64	3.99	
Guideline	600	2.0	.015	.120	11.40	3.75	
Conclusion	*	[]	N.K.	*	*	*	*

Elevated fat level. Not recommended.

Morning Sun Natural Apricot and Almond Muesli

Advertising claim: "No added salt. Cholesterol free"

Food Factor	Energy	Fat	Cholest.	Sodium	Sugar	Fibre
Labelling	1470	8.0	N.S	.0326	19.3	12.3
As consumed with						
milk only	573	2.66	N.K.	.046	9.64	3.99
Guideline	600	2.0	.015	.120	11.40	3.75
Conclusion	*	[]	N.K.	*	*	*

Elevated fat level. Not recommended.

Purina Swiss Formula Muesli

Food Factor	Energy	Fat	Cholest.	Sodium	Sugar	Fibre	Addit.
Labelling	1380	7.8	Nil	.019	17	14.4	None
As consumed with							
milk only	544	2.59	.001	.041	8.89	4.67	
Guideline	600	2.0	.015	.120	11.40	3.75	
Conclusion	*	[]	*	*	*	*	*

*Despite a largely excellent low-risk profile, elevated fat level.
Not recommended.*

Farmland No Added Salt Tropical Toasted Muesli with Six Fruits

Food Factor	Energy	Fat	Cholest.	Sodium	Sugar	Fibre	Addit.
Labelling	1730	14	N.S.	.030	19	2	None
As consumed with							
milk only	657	8.53	N.K.	.045	9.54	.65	
Guideline	600	2.0	.015	.120	11.40	3.75	
Conclusion	[ ]	[ ]	N.K.	*	*	N.A.	*

Elevated fat level. Not recommended.

Goodness Products Tropical Fruits Toasted Muesli

Advertising claim: "No added salt. one-third less fat; N.H.F. approved"

Food Factor	Energy	Fat	Cholest.	Sodium	Sugar	Fibre	Addit.
Labelling	1569	8.7	N.S.	.009	15.4	7.4	None
As consumed with							
milk only	633	2.81	N.K.	.037	10.75	2.34	
Guideline	600	2.0	.015	.120	11.40	3.75	
Conclusion	=	[ ]	N.K.	*	*	N.A.	*

Borderline energy level and elevated fat level. Not recommended.

Morning Sun Toasted Tropical Fruits Muesli

Advertising claim: "No added salt"

Food Factor	Energy	Fat	Cholest.	Sodium	Sugar	Fibre
Labelling	1650	13.6	N.S.	.028	16.4	7.6
As consumed with						
milk only	658	4.36	N.K.	.045	11.1	2.4
Guideline	600	2.0	.015	.120	11.40	3.75
Conclusion	[ ]		[ ]	N.K.	*	*	N.A.

Additive Code.	471	433
Translation	Fatty acid diglycerides	Polysorbate
Function	Emulsifier	Emulsifier
Conclusion	*	*

Elevated fat level. Not recommended.

Best Foods White Wings Nature Valley Toasted Muesli Flakes

Food Factor	Energy	Fat	Cholest.	Sodium	Sugar	Fibre
Labelling		2.5	N.S.	N.S.	17.5	7.5
As consumed with						
milk only	580	.855	N.K.	N.K.	11.97	2.37
Guideline	600	2.0	.015	.120	11.40	3.75
Conclusion	*	*	N.K.	N.K.	=	N.A.

Additive Code	330
Translation	Citric acid
Function	Food acid
Conclusion	*

*An unusual nutritional panel, providing all the usual data —
except for sodium. As this is the key risk-factor for cereals,
and 'salt added' is noted on the ingredients list — not
recommended.*

7

Breads, biscuits and cakes

Conventional bread is above guidelines in energy and sodium. The sodium level can easily be reduced, and low sodium breads are increasingly available. This is important, as breads and cereals are the major sources of excess sodium in the Australian diet[44].

The energy issue is harder to address. Breads are high energy foods because they are made from a material -- wheat seeds -- which Nature has dried for storage. And the amount of water added in the making of bread does not 'dilute' flour to the same extent that, say, milk dilutes breakfast cereal.

Because of the fact that the energy level of even the lowest energy breads is above guideline, bread is recommended for use, but not as freely as other starch sources such as potatoes (which, with their higher water content) are within the energy guideline.

For biscuits and cakes, the potential risk factors include levels of fat and sugars as well as sodium and energy.

Sunicrust Suni Sandwich Wholemeal Bread

Advertising claim: "Low in calories, fat and cholesterol"

Food Factor	Energy	Fat	Cholest.	Sodium	Sugar	Fibre
Labelling	884	2.2	N.S.	.510	2.0	5.8
Guideline	600	2.0	.015	.120	5.0	3.75
Conclusion	[ ]	=	N.K.	[ ]	*	*

Additive Code	471		262	281
Translation	Fatty acid glycerides		Sodium diacetate	Sodium propionate
Function	Stabiliser	Preservative	Preservative	
Conclusion	*		*	see Appendix I

Elevated energy and sodium. Not recommended.

Buttercup Gold Medal Oat Bran Bread

Food Factor	Energy	Fat	Cholest.	Sodium	Sugar	Fibre
Labelling	950	3.0	N.S.	.380	2.0	8.60
Guideline	600	2.0	.015	.120	5.0	3.75
Conclusion	[ ]	[ ]	N.K.	[ ]	*	*

Additive Code	471	472(e)
Translation	Fatty acid glycerides	Glycerol esters
Function	Stabiliser	Stabiliser
Conclusion	*	*

Elevated in energy and sodium. Not recommended.

Buttercup Natural Grain Toasting Bread

Advertising claim: "1/3 less salt"

Food Factor	Energy	Fat	Cholest.	Sodium	Sugar	Fibre	Addit.
Labelling	982	3.2	N.S.	.331	2.6	1.1	None
Guideline	600	2.0	.015	.120	5.0	3.75	
Conclusion	[]	[]	N.K.	[]	*	N.A.	*

Salt reduction insufficient to bring within guideline. Fat and energy also elevated. Not recommended.

Naturlich Protein Increased Wholemeal Bread

Advertising claim: "No sugar, shortening, cholesterol. Low salt"

Food Factor	Energy	Fat	Cholest.	Sodium	Sugar	Fibre
Labelling	90.0	2.0	N.S.	.150	1.5	6.0
Guideline	600	2.0	.015	.120	5.0	3.75
Conclusion	[]	=	N.K.	[]	*	*

Additive Code	508	472(e)
Translation	Potassium chloride	Glycerol esters
Function	Salt substitute	Stabiliser
Conclusion	*	*

Elevated energy. Sodium, although markedly reduced on normal bread, also still above guideline. Not recommended.

Riga Pritikin Bread

*Advertising claim: "No shortening or other fat added; no
artificial colours or flavours; low salt"*

Food Factor	Energy	Fat	Cholest.	Sodium	Sugar	Fibre	Addit.
Labelling	956	1.6	0	.017	< 2	8	None
Guideline	600	2.0	.015	.120	5.0	3.75	
Conclusion	[ ]	*	*	*	*	*	*

*Except for energy level (which is that of average wholemeal
bread), a straight star profile. For use in moderation,
recommended.*

Country Bake True Traditional Sliced White Bread

*Advertising claim: "No preservatives, no artificial colours,
flavours or emulsifiers"*

Food Factor	Energy	Fat	Cholest.	Sodium	Sugar	Fibre	Addit.
Labelling	940	2.3	0	.510	1.0	N.S.	None
Guideline	600	2.0	.015	.120	5.0	3.75	
Conclusion	[ ]	=	*	[ ]	*	N.A	*.

Elevated sodium level, as well as energy. Not recommended.

Vogel's Stoneground Wholemeal and Sesame Bread

Food Factor	Energy	Fat	Cholest.	Sodium	Sugar	Fibre	Addit.
Labelling	1055	5.9	N.S.	.550	2.7	1.2	None
Guideline	600	2.0	.015	.120	5.0	3.75	
Conclusion	[ ]		[ ]	N.K.	[ ]	*	*	*

SUMMARY Sesame seed content markedly elevates fat level and hence energy content of this bread. Sodium also well above guideline. Not recommended.

Vogel's Original Mixed Grain Bread

Food Factor	Energy	Fat	Cholest.	Sodium	Sugar	Fibre	Addit.
Labelling	990	2.6	N.S.	.470	3.0	5.5	None
Guideline	600	2.0	.015	.120	5.0	3.75	
Conclusion	[ ]		[ ]	N.K.	[ ]	*	*	*

Above guideline fat, sodium and energy. Not recommended.

Regal Oat'n'Bran Bread

Food Factor	Energy	Fat	Cholest.	Sodium	Sugar	Fibre	Addit.
Labelling	925	2.0	N.S.	.380	2.0	4.0	None
Guideline	600	2.0	.015	.120	5.0	3.75	
Conclusion	[ ]		*	N.K.	[ ]	*	*	*

Above guideline sodium and energy. Not recommended.

Cereal Foods Premium Lite Crispbread

Advertising claim: "Only 56 Kilojoules per slice"

Food Factor	Energy	Fat	Cholest.	Sodium	Sugar	Fibre
Labelling	1542	11.8	N.S.	N.S.	N.S.	1.45
Guideline	600	2.0	.015	.120	5.0	3.75
Conclusion	*	*	N.K.	N.K.	N.K.	[ ]

Additive Code	500		481		471
Translation	Sodium sesauicarbonate		Sodium stearoyl lactylate		Mono-diglyceride
Function	Acidity adjuster		both consistency enhancers		
Conclusion	*		*		*

Above guidelines for energy and fat. Not recommended,

Vogel's Swiss Style Mixed Grain Bread   Now with Oat Bran

Advertising claim: "Now with oat bran; 1/3 less salt than most other breads"

Food Factor	Energy	Fat	Cholest.	Sodium	Sugar	Fibre	Addit.
Labelling	1000	2.8	N.S.	.240	2.3	5.5	None
Guideline	600	2.0	.015	.120	5.0	3.75	
Conclusion	[ ]	[ ]	N.K.	[ ]	*	*	*

Above guidelines for energy, fat and sodium. Not recommended.

Cereal Foods 50% Less Salt Premium Crackers

Food Factor	Energy	Fat	Cholest.	Sodium	Sugar	Fibre
Labelling	1910	17.4	N.S.	.440	2.0	N.S.
Guideline	600	2.0	.015	.120	5.0	3.75
Conclusion	[ ]		[ ]	N.K.	[ ]	*	N.K.

Additive Code	500
Translation	Sodium sesquicarbonate
Function	Acidity adjuster
Conclusion	*

Outside guidelines in fat, energy and — despite reduction — sodium. Not recommended.

Willow Valley Crispbread with Oat Bran

Advertising claim: "Recommended by Fiona Coote"

Food Factor	Energy	Fat	Cholest.	Sodium	Sugar	Fibre	Addit.
Labelling	1430	3.4	N.S.	.299	N.S.	7.5	None
Guideline	600	2.0	.015	.120	5.0	3.75	
Conclusion	[ ]	[ ]	N.K.	[ ]	N.K.	*	*

Elevated energy, fat and sodium. Not recommended.

Ryvita No Added Salt Whole Rye Crispbread

Food Factor	Energy	Fat	Cholest.	Sodium	Sugar	Fibre	Addit.
Labelling	1310	2.0	N.S.	.001	appr.3	14.9	None
Guideline	600	2.0	.015	.120	5.0	3.75	
Conclusion	[ ]	=	N.K.	*	*	*	*

Except for energy content, an otherwise low-risk profile. For this reason, recommended for sparing use.

Westons Oatcrisps Crispbread

*Advertising claim: "Good food in a snack: only 127Kj per
bite-sized piece"*

Food Factor	Energy	Fat	Cholest.	Sodium	Sugar	Fibre	Addit.
Labelling	1498	4.2	N.S.	.385	6.5	.4.3	None
Guideline	600	2.0	.015	.120	5.0	3.75	
Conclusion	[ ]	[ ]	N.K.	[ ]	*	*	*

*Despite implications of slogan, repeatedly outside our
guidelines. Not recommended.*

Limmits Calorie Controlled Meal Replacement Chocolate Valencia Meals

Food Factor	Energy	Fat	Cholest.	Sodium	Sugar	Fibre
Labelling	2019	26	N.S.	.300	55	5
Guideline	600	2.0	.015	.120	11.40	3.75
Conclusion	[ ]	[ ]	N.K.	[ ]	[ ]	*

Additive Code	412	102	110	150
Translation	Guar gum	Tartrazine	Sunset Yellow	Caramel
Function	Thickener	Colour	Colour	Colour
Conclusion		see Appendix I	see Appendix I	see Appendix I

Additive Code	330	310	320
Translation	Citric acid	Propyl gallate	Butylated hydroxyanisole
Function	Food acid	both Antioxidants (preservatives)	
Conclusion	*	see Appendix I	

*Repeatedly and markedly above guidelines. Not
recommended.*

Limmits Calorie Controlled Meal Replacement Cheese'n'Chives Sandwich Meal

Food Factor	Energy	Fat	Cholest.	Sodium	Sugar	Fibre
Labelling	2140	30	N.S.	.680	53	4.5
Guideline	600	2.0	.015	.120	5.0	3.75
Conclusion	[ ]	[ ]	N.K.	[ ]	[ ]	*

Additive Code	412	621	310	320
Translation	Guar gum	MSG	Propyl gallate	Butylated, Hydroxy anisole
Function	Thickener	Flavour enhancer	both Antioxidants (preservatives)	
Conclusion	*	see Appendix I	see Appendix I	

Repeatedly outside guidelines. Not recommended.

Sara Lee Hearty Fruit Muffins (Blueberry)

	Energy	Fat	Cholest.	Sodium	Sugar	Fibre	Addit.
Labelling	1370	14.9	N.S.	.340	23.6	N.S	None
Guideline	6,00	2.0	.015	.120	11.40	3.75	
Conclusion	[ ]	[ ]	N.K.	[ ]	[ ]	N.K.	*

Numerous above-guideline food factors. Not recommended.

Arrowhead Mills Oat Bran Pancake and Waffle Mix

Food Factor	Energy	Fat	Cholest.	Sodium	Sugar	Fibre	Addit.
Labelling	1499	3.57	N.S	.409	N.S.	N.S.	None
Guideline	600	2.0	.015	.120	5.0	3.75	
Conclusion	[ ]	[ ]	N.K.	[ ]	N.K.	N.A.	*

Elevated in energy, fat and sodium. Not recommended.

Arrowhead Mills Apple and Spice Oatbran Muffin Mix

Food Factor	Energy	Fat	Cholest.	Sodium	Sugar	Fibre
Labelling	1499	7.14	N.S	.620	N.S.	N.S.
Guideline	600	2.0	.015	.120	11.40	3.75
Conclusion	[ ]	[ ]	N.K.	[ ]	N.K.	N.A.

Additive Code 415

Translation	Xanthan gum
Function	Thickener
Conclusion	*

Fat and sodium markedly above guidelines. Not recommended.

Clarke's Apricot Bran Cookies

Advertising claim: "All natural"

Food Factor	Energy	Fat	Cholest.	Sodium	Sugar	Fibre	Addit.
Labelling	1887	18.9	0	.246	22.5	7.52	None
Guideline	600	.2.0	.015	.120	11.40	3.75	
Conclusion	[]	[]	*	[]	[]	*	*

Despite good fibre level, other food components above guidelines. Not recommended.

Uncle Toby's Oat Bran Muffin Mix with Sultanas and Almonds

Advertising claim: "Can help reduce cholesterol (when part of a low fat, low cholesterol diet)"

Food Factor	Energy	Fat	Cholest.	Sodium	Sugars	Fibre		Addit.
							Total Sol.	
Labelling	1560	12.6	0	.561	27.9	10.7	4.2	None
Guideline	600	2.0	.015	.120	11.40	3.75	1.8	
Conclusion	[]	[]	*	[]	[]	*	*	*

A good source of fibre, but outside guidelines for fat, sodium, sugars and energy. Not recommended.

Uncle Toby's Rice Bran Muffin Mix

Food Factor	Energy	Fat	Cholest.	Sodium	Sugar	Fibre	Addit.
Labelling	1580	13.8	Nil	.378	24.7	10.8	None
Guideline	600	2.0	.015	.120	11.40	3.75	
Conclusion	[]	[]	*	[]	[]	*	*

Several elevated food components. Not recommended.

Clarke's Raisin and Sesame Low Cholesterol Cookies – Now with added Oat Bran

Advertising claim: "Never before has anyone combined taste and nutrition so deliciously"

Food Factor	Energy	Fat	Cholest.	Sodium	Sugar	Fibre	Addit.
Labelling	2297	38.5	N.S	.376	19.0	6.1	None
Guideline	600	2.0	.015	.120	11.40	3.75	
Conclusion	[ ]	[ ]	N.K.	[ ]	[ ]	*	*

Food components repeatedly outside guidelines. Not recommended.

Willow Valley Chewy Oat Bran Cookies with Fruit and Nuts

Food Factor	Energy	Fat	Cholest.	Sodium	Sugar	Fibre	Addit.
Labelling	1958	23.34	0	.201	42.2	5.37	None
Guideline	600	2.0	.015	.120	11.40	3.75	
Conclusion	[ ]	[ ]	*	[ ]	[ ]	*	*

Several above guideline food components. Not recommended.

Only Natural Organically Grown Rice Cakes

Advertising claim: "Cholesterol free"

Food Factor	Energy	Fat	Cholest.	Sodium	Sugar	Fibre	Addit.
Labelling	1540	2.0	0	.004	0.4	3.2	None
Guideline	600	2.0	.015	.120	5.0	3.75	
Conclusion	[ ]	*	*	*	*	=	*

All food components within guidelines except energy. Recommended for sparing use.

Naturally Good Peanut Crunch Cookies

Advertising claim: "Dairy, wheat and gluten free.; low cholesterol, low salt"

Food Factor	Energy	Fat	Cholest.	Sodium	Sugar	Fibre	Addit.
Labelling	2169	30.0	.005	.016	29.0	N.S.	None
Guideline	600	2.0	.015	.120	11.4	3.75	
Conclusion	[]	[]	*	*	[]	N.A.	*

Markedly above guidelines for energy, fat and sugars. Not recommended.

8

Spreads

Spreads for bread tend to be concentrated food products. However, the key issue is their effect on food intakes as consumed. In what follows, we assess spreads as optimally consumed, 5g spread alone on 45g no-added-salt bread.

Conventional Peanut Butter

Food Factor	Energy	Fat	Cholest.	Sodium	Sugar	Fibre	Addit.
Content	2581	53.7	0	.350	6.7	7.6.	None
As consumed on bread	1102	7.76	0	.080	3.69	8.4	
Guideline	600	2.0	.015	.120	5.0	3.75	
Conclusion	[ ]	[ ]	*	*	*	*	*

Conventional (salted) peanut butter is within sodium guideline after 'dilution' as consumed spread on no-added-salt bread. But, even as consumed, peanut butter is still elevated in fat and energy. For special occasions only.

Unsalted Peanut Butter

Food Facts	Energy	Fat	Cholest.	Sodium	Sugar	Fibre	Addit.
content	2581	53.7	0	.006	6.7	7.6.	None
As consumed on bread	1102	7.76	0	.029	3.69	8.4	
Guideline	600	2.0	.015	.120	5.0	3.75	
Conclusion	[ ]	[ ]	*	*	*	*	*

Elevated in energy and fat. For special occasions only.

Honey

Food Factor	Energy	Fat	Cholest.	Sodium	Sugar	Fibre	Addit.
Content	1201	0	0	.007	74.4	0	None
As consumed on bread	949	1.78	0	.031	11.42	7.6	
Guideline	600	2.0	.015	.120	11.4	3.75	
Conclusion	[ ]	*	*	*	*	*	*

As consumed on bread, only energy is above guideline. Recommended for moderate use.

Conventional Jam (Blackberry)

Food Factor	Energy	Fat	Cholest.	Sodium	Sugar	Fibre	Addit.
Content	1114	0	0	.016	69.0	1.1	None
As consumed							
on bread	940	1.78	0	.031	10.69	7.7	
Guideline	600	2.0	.015	.120	5.0	3.75	
Conclusion	[ ]	*	*	*	*	*	*

Except for energy (and this mainly from bread, not jam), a straight within-guideline profile. For use in moderation, recommended.

Weight Watchers Low Joule Apricot Jam

Advertising claim: "50% more fruit than standard jams"

Food Factor	Energy	Fat	Cholest.	Sodium	Sugar	Fibre
Labelling	130		0	.144	7.9	N.S.
As consumed						
on bread	831	1.78	0	.051	3.82	7.6
Guideline	6 0 0	2.0	.015	.120	11.40	3 . 7 5
Conclusion	[ ]	*	*	*	*	*

Additive Code	407	410		330
Translation	Irish moss	Carob bean gum	Cyclamate	Citric acid
Function	Thickener	Thickener	Artificial sweetener	Setting agent
Conclusion	*	*	see Appendix I *	

Additive Code	332	211	160(a) & 160(e)
Translation	Potassium dihydrogen citrate	Sodium benzoate	Carotenes
Function.	Emulsifier	Preservative	Colours
Conclusion	*	see Appendix I	*

As consumed, all food components within guidelines except energy (which is due to bread). But so are results from orthodox jams, which are without the additives. Not really recommended.

Sanitarium Yeast Extract — Marmite

Food Factor	Energy	Fat	Cholest.	Sodium	Sugar	Fibre	Addit.
Content	837	.5	0	4.400	5.2	N.S.	None
As consumed on bread	909	1.83	.0	.504	3.51	7.6	
Guideline	600	2.0	.015	.120	5.0	3.75	
Conclusion	[ ]	*	*	[ ]	*	*	*

Elevated in energy (because bread itself is). But even after dilution to a tenth, the sodium level of bread and Marmite remains markedly above guidelines. Not recommended.

Flora Light — Polyunsaturated Reduced Fat Spread

Advertising claim: "39% less fat. Salt reduced; N.H.F. approved"

Food Factor	Energy	Fat	Cholest.	Sodium	Sugar	Fibre
Labelling	1850	49	N.S.	.391	.35	N.S. (0)
As consumed on bread	1060	7.0	0	.060	3.00	7.6
Guideline	600	2.0	.015	.120	5.0	3.75
Conclusion	[ ]	[ ]	N.K.	*	*	*

Additive Code	322	202	270	160(b)	100
Translation	Lecithin	Potassium sorbate	Lactic acid	Annatto	Curcumin
Function	Emulsifier	Preservat.	Anti-oxidant	Colour	Colour
Conclusion	*	*	*	*	*

Fat reduction still does not bring bread and margarine within our guidelines. Despite National Heart Foundation approval, not recommended.

Era Polyunsaturated Reduced Fat Spread with Buttermilk

Advertising claim: "Half the fat . . . cholesterol free"

Food Factor	Energy	Fat	Cholest.	Sodium	Sugar	Fibre
Labelling	1600	40	0	.200	.28	N.A.
As consumed on bread	993	6.2	0	.038	2.96	7.6
Guideline	600	2.0	.015	.120	5.0	3.75
Conclusion	[ ]	[ ]	*	*	*	*

Additive Code	471		322	270		202
Translation	Mono-/di-glycerides		Lecithin	Lactic acid		Potassium sorbate
Function	Emulsifier		Emulsifier	Antioxidant		Preservative
Conclusion	*		*	*		*

Additive Code	160(a)
Translation	Beta carotene
Function	Yellow colour
Conclusion	*

Marked reduction in fat and energy over conventional margarines, but even as consumed, still above guidelines. Not recommended.

Becel Light

Advertising claim: "Cholesterol free; Salt free; Milk free; N.H.F. approved"

Food Factor	Energy	Fat	Cholest.	Sodium	Sugar	Fibre
Labelling	1480	40.0	Nil	Nil	Nil	N.S
As consumed						
on bread	920	6.2	0	.030	2.6	7.6
Guideline	600	2.0	.015	.120	5.0	3.75
Conclusion	[ ]	[ ]	*	*	*	*

Additive Code	322	202		270	160(a)
Translation	Lecithin	Potassium sorbate		Lactic acid	Beta carotene
Function	Emulsifier	Preservative		Antioxidant	Colour
Conclusion	*	*		*	*

Additive Code	471
Translation	mono-/di-glycerides
Function	Emulsifiers
Conclusion	*

Fat and energy above guidelines despite fat reduction. Not recommended.

Farmland Salt Free Milk Free Cholesterol Free Polyunsaturated Margarine

Food Factor	Energy	Fat	Cholest.	Sodium	Sugar	Fibre
Labelling	3115	83.7	Nil	Nil	Nil	N.S.
As consumed on bread	1160	10.8	0	.030	2.6	7.6
Guideline	600	2.0		.120	5.0	3.75
Conclusion	[ ]	[ ]	*	*	*	*

Additive Code	322	16O(a)	471
Translation	Lecithin	Beta carotene	Mono-/di-glycerides
Function	Emulsifier	Colour	Emulsifiers
Conclusion	*	*	*

Energy and fat elevated. Not recommended.

Weight Watchers Whipped Polyunsaturated Margarine

Advertising claim: "Contains less than 5mg Cholesterol per 100g"

Food Factor	Energy	Fat	Cholest.	Sodium	Sugar	Fibre
Labelling	3020	81.3	.005	N.S.	N.S.(O)	N.S.
As consumed on bread	1160	11.0	.005	N.K.	2.6	7.6
Guideline	600	2.0	.015	.120	5.0	3.75
Conclusion	[ ]	[ ]	*	N.K.	*	*

Additive Code	322	160(a)	471
Translation	Lecithin	Beta carotene	Mono-/di-glycerides
Function	Emulsifier	Colour	Emulsifiers
Conclusion	*	*	*

Elevated fat and energy. Not recommended.

<u>INDEPENDENT LABORATORY TEST</u>

Modern Health Products Natex Yeast Extract

Food Factor	Energy	Fat	Cholest.	Sodium	Sugar	Fibre	Addit.
Labelling	910	.1	N.S.(O)	.400	.3	N.S.	None
Test				.310			
As consumed	891	1.79	0	.051	3.02	7.56	
Guideline	600	2.0	.015	.120	5.0	3.75	
Conclusion	[ ]	*	*	*	*	*	*

Except for energy (due to bread), an all star profile.
Recommended.

<u>INDEPENDENT LABORATORY TEST</u>

The Island Fruit Company Australian Natural Salt Reduced Savoury Yeast Extract

Food Factor	Energy	Fat	Cholest.	Sodium	Sugar	Fibre	Addit.
Labelling	N.S.	N.S.	N.S.	N.S.	N.S.	N.S.	None
	(687)	(O)	(O)		(11.8)	(O)	
Test				1.100			
As consumed	891	1.78	0	.138	4.24	7.56	
Guideline	600	2.0	.015	.120	5.0	3.75	
Conclusion	[ ]	*	*	=	*	*	*

No labelling is provided for this claimed salt-reduced spread,
so figures in brackets are for typical values for yeast extracts.
We independently tested the key food component concerning
yeast extracts, sodium.
Energy outside guidelines (due to bread). All other factors
within guidelines but sodium, which is borderline, but
nonetheless a marked improvement over conventional yeast
extracts. For this reason, recommended.Note, however, that
another yeast extract, Natex has a well <u>within</u> guideline
sodium level.

Holiday Isle New Formula Cholesterol Free, Milk Free, Salt Reduced Margarine

Food Factor	Energy	Fat	Cholest.	Sodium	Sugar	Fibre
Labelling	3000	80.0	0	.400	1.2	N.S.
As consumed on bread	1149	10.7	0	.060	3.02	7.6
Guideline	600	2.0	.015	.120	5.0	3.75
Conclusion	[]	[]	*	*	*	*

Additive Code	322	160(a)	471
Translation	Lecithin	Beta carotene	Monodiglycerides
Function	Emulsifier	Colour	Emulsifiers
Conclusion	*	*	*

Elevated fat, even as consumed. Not recommended.

Nuttelex Polyunsaturated Margarine

Advertising claim: "Milk free, salt reduced. Cholesterol free"

Food Factor	Energy	Fat	Cholest.	Sodium	Sugar	Fibre
Labelling	3000	83	Nil	.600	Nil	N.A.
As consumed on bread	1149	11.0	0	.070	2.6	7.6
Guideline	600	2.0	.015	.120	5.0	3.75
Conclusion	[]	[]	*	*	*	*

Additive Code	322	471
Translation	Lecithin	Mono-/di-glycerides
Function	Emulsifier	Emulsifiers
Conclusion	*	*

Energy and fat above guidelines. Not recommended.

Gold'n Canola Salt Reduced Margarine
(Meadow Lea)

Advertising claim: "Fight cholesterol; N.H.F. approved"

Food Factor	Energy	Fat	Cholest.	Sodium	Sugar	Fibre
Labelling	3049	82.0	Nil	.393	.51	N.S.
As consumed						
on bread	1151	10.8	0	.059	2.98	7.60
Guideline	600	2.0	.015	.120	5.0	3.75
Conclusion	[ ]	[ ]	*	*	*	*

Additive Code	322	160(a)	471
Translation	Lecithin	Beta carotene	Mono-/di-glycerides
Function	Emulsifier	Colour	Emulsifiers
Conclusion	*	*	*

Energy and fat elevated. Not recommended.

9

Cheeses

It is almost easier for the camel to pass through the eye of the needle than it is for one to find a cheese which is within our guidelines. This is because cheese is a highly concentrated food, generally elevated in energy, fat, cholesterol and sodium.

Recognising this, the dairy industry have been producing a wide range of products claiming reductions in levels of one or more of these food factors, and a number of these new products are included in the cheeses reviewed in this chapter.

McMahon's Low Salt Reduced Fat Cheddar Cheese

Food Factor	Energy	Fat	Cholest.	Sodium	Sugar	Fibre	Addit.
Labelling	N.S.	<24.0	N.S.	<.121	N.S.	N.S.	None
Guideline	600	2.0	.015	.120	5.0	3.75	
Conclusion	N.K.	[ ]	N.K.	*	N.K.	N.K.	*

The salt reduction is welcome, but with fat above the guideline and energy and cholesterol likely to be, not recommended.

Kraft Light Philadelphia Smooth Blend of Cream Cheese and Cottage Cheese

Advertising claim: "82% Fat Free"

Food Factor	Energy	Fat	Cholest.	Sodium	Sugar	Fibre
Labelling	820	16.5	.095	.340	3.1	*N.S.*
Guideline	600	2.0	.015	.120	5.0	3.75
Conclusion	[ ]	[ ]	[ ]	[ ]	*	N.A.

Additive Code	412
Translation	Guar gum
Function	Thickener
Conclusion	*

Despite reductions in fat and sodium levels, food components are generally elevated above guidelines. Not recommended.

Kraft Light Cheese Spread — A Blend of Cheddar and Cottage Cheese Spread

Advertising claim: "50% less cholesterol than most natural cheddar cheeses"

Food Factor	Energy	Fat	Cholest.	Sodium	Sugar	Fibre
Labelling	1080	17	.052	1.290	4.6	Nil
Guideline	600	2.0	.015	.120	5.0	3.75
Conclusion	[ ]	[ ]	[ ]	[ ]	*	N.A.

Additive Code	339		450	270
Translation	Sodium phosphate		Potassium polyphosphate	Lactic acid
Function	Texture improver		Stabiliser	Preservative
Conclusion	see Appendix I		see Appendix I	*

Additive Code	200	160(b)	
Translation	Sorbic acid	Annatto	Retinol (Vitamin A)
Function	Preservative	Colour	Fortifier
Conclusion	*	*	*

Despite a fat reduction, still above the guideline for fat, and for several other food components. Not recommended.

Bega Super Slims

Advertising claim: "50% less fat than normal processed cheese"

Food Factor	Energy	Fat	Cholest.	Sodium	Sugar	Fibre
Labelling	983	11.0	N.S.	1.435	N.S.(O)	Nil
Guideline	600	2.0	.015	.120	5.0	3.75
Conclusion	[ ]	[ ]	N.K.	[ ]	*	N.A.

Additive Code	331	260
Translation	Sodium citrates	Acetic acid
Function	Antioxidant	Stabiliser
Conclusion	*	*

Substantial fat reductions, but fat (and other components) still above guidelines. Not recommended.

Coon Light Reduced Fat Cheddar Cheese

Advertising claim: "20% reduced fat and cholesterol"

Food Factor	Energy	Fat	Cholest.	Sodium	Sugar	Fibre	Addit.
Labelling	1472	26	.800	.770	<1	Nil	None
Guideline	600	2.0	.015	.120	5.0	3.75	
Conclusion	[ ]	[ ]	[ ]	[ ]	*	N.A.	*

Although indeed reduced in fat, still markedly above fat guideline, as well as several others. Not recommended.

Western Star Reduced Fat Processed Cheese Slices

Food Factor	Energy	Fat	Cholest.	Sodium	Sugar	Fibre
Labelling	983	11.0	N.S. (.070)	1.435	2	Nil
Guideline	600	2.0	.015	.120	5.0	3.75
Conclusion	[ ]	[ ]	([ ])	[ ]	*	N.A.

Additive Code	331	260
Translation	Sodium citrates	Acetic acid
Function	Antioxidant	Stabiliser
Conclusion	*	*

Relatively large fat reduction for a cheddar-style cheese, but still outside guideline. And, surprisingly for a health-oriented product, sodium level is higher than for normal cheddars! Not recommended.

Bega So Light -- 25% Reduced Fat Cheddar

Food Factor	Energy	Fat	Cholest.	Sodium	Sugar	Fibre	Addit.
Labelling	1450	26	N.S. (.070)	.610	Nil	N.S.	None
Guideline	600	2.0	.015 .	120	5.0	3.75	
Conclusion	[ ]	[ ]	([ ])	[ ]	*	N.A.	*

Above guidelines for several food components. Not recommended.

Kraft Light Slices

Advertising claim: "30% less fat than processed cheese slices"

Food Factor	Energy	Fat	Cholest.	Sodium	Sugar	Fibre
Labelling	1078	16.5	N.S. (.070)	1.275	4	N.S.
Guideline	600	2.0	.015	.120	5.0	3.75
Conclusion	[ ]	[ ]	([ ])	[ ]	*	N.A.

Additive Code	339		508	270	200
Translation	Sodium phosphate		Potassium chloride	Lactic acid	Sorbic acid
Function	Stabiliser		Salt substitute	Preservative	Preservative
Conclusion	see Appendix I	see Appendix I		*	*

Additive Code	331
Translation	Sodium citrates
Function	Preservative
Conclusion	*

Less fat, but still above guidelines for fat, and for other components. Not recommended.

Devondale Moo Squares

Advertising claim: "15% fat, 25% less salt"

Food Factor	Energy	Fat	Cholest.	Sodium	Sugar	Fibre
Labelling	1081	15.0	N.S. (.070)	1.100	1.0	N.S.
Guideline	600	2.0	.015	.120	5.0	3.75
Conclusion	[]	[]	([])	[]	*	N.A.

Additive Code	331	339
Translation	Sodium citrates	Sodium phosphate
Function	Preservative	Stabiliser
Conclusion	*	see Appendix I

Despite substantial fat reduction and some sodium reduction, still well above Guidelines. Not recommended.

Bulla Low Fat Cottage Cheese with Pineapple

Food Factor	Energy	Fat	Cholest.	Sodium	Sugar	Fibre
Labelling	387	1.5	.015	.310	8.7	N.S.
Guideline	600	2.0	.015	.120	11.4	3.75
Conclusion	*	*	*	[]	*	N.A.

Additive Code	330	202
Translation	Citric acid	Potassium sorbate
Function	Food acid	Preservative
Conclusion	*	*

A generally within-guideline profile. But because of the sodium level, not recommended.

Quark Low Fat Cheese
(general type) (Source: dairy industry data)

Food factor	Energy	Fat	Cholest.	Sodium	Sugar	Fibre	Addit.
Labelling	315	0.2	.010	.160	2.9	N.S. (0)	None
Guideline	600	2.0	.015	.120	5.0	3.75	
Conclusion	*	*	*	[ ]	*	N.A.	*

All food factors but sodium are within guidelines, and sodium is only slightly elevated. Recommended for use as 50% or less of otherwise very low sodium dish.

Cotto Cheese
(general type) (Source: dairy industry data)

Food Factor	Energy	Fat	Cholest.	Sodium	Sugar	Fibre	Addit.
Labelling	885	11.0.	.050	.750	0.5	N.S.(0)	None
Guideline	600	2.0	.015	.120	5.0	3.75	
Conclusion	[ ]	[ ]	[ ]	[ ]	*	N.A.	*

Many elevated food factors. Not recommended.

<u>**INDEPENDENT LABORATORY TEST**</u>

Devondale Seven Full Flavour Cheese

Advertising claim: "Low fat, low cholesterol"

Food Factor	Energy	Fat	Cholest.	Sodium	Sugar	Fibre	Addit.
Labelling	807	7.0	.038	.500	<.1	Nil	None
Test	6.5						
Guideline	600	2.0	.015	.120	5.0	3.75	
Conclusion	[ ]	[ ]	[ ]	[ ]	*	N.A.	*

This new cheddar-style cheese claims a marked (almost 80 per cent) reduction in fat over conventional cheddar. As such, it represents an important step towards healthier cheeses. For this reason, we independently laboratory tested the fat level. The result showed a figure of 6.5g/100g, confirming the 7g/100g labelling claim.

However, the table shows that even despite the fat reduction, and a lower than average sodium level, Devondale Seven is still outside most of our guidelines. Nonetheless, because it has by far the best overall profile of any cheddar-type cheese, it is conditionally recommended for use in meals -- as <u>one-fifth or less</u> of otherwise within guideline dishes.

Perfect Cheese Smooth Ricotta Cheese Spread

Food Factor	Energy	Fat	Cholest.	Sodium	Sugar	Fibre
Labelling	420	7.0	N.S.(.15)	.130	3.2	N.S.
As consumed	862	2.56	.002	.030	3.29	7.56
Guideline	600	2.0	.015	.120	5.0	3.75
Conclusion	*	[ ]	*	*	*	*

Additive Code	202
Translation	Potassium sorbate
Function	preservative
Conclusion	*

Even as consumed on bread, fat level is above guidelines. Not recommended.

Bodalla Reduced Fat and Salt Cheddar Cheese

Food Factor	Energy	Fat	Cholest.	Sodium	Sugar	Fibre	Addit.
Labelling	1455	25.1	N.S. (.070)	.300	.05	*N.S.*	None
Guideline	600	2.0	.015	.12 0	5.0	3.75	
Conclusion	[ ]	[ ]	[ ]	[ ]	*	N.A.	*

Despite some reduction in fat and sodium, these and other food components are still well outside guidelines. Not recommended.

Kraft Reduced Fat Mozarella Shredded Cheese

Advertising claim: "20% less fat (not more than 19% fat)"

Food Factor	Energy	Fat	Cholest.	Sodium	Sugar	Fibre	Addit.
Labelling	N.S.	19.0	N.S.	N.S.	N.S.	N.S.	None
Guideline	600	2.0	.015	.120	5.0	3.75	
Conclusion	N.K.	[ ]	N.K	N.K.	N.K.	N.A.	*

Fat level still well above guideline. Not recommended.

Meadow Gold Creamed Cottage Cheese (Reduced Salt)

Advertising claim: "Reduced salt: 0.45%. Milk fat 4%"

Food Factor	Energy	Fat	Cholest.	Sodium	Sugar	Fibre	Addit.
Labelling	N.S.	4.0	N.S.	.180	N.S.	N.S.	None
Guideline	600	2.0	.015	.120	5.0	3.75	
Conclusion	N.K.	[ ]	N.K.	[ ]	N.K.	N.A.	*

Reduced salt products generally do not fall within low salt guidelines, and Meadow Gold is no exception. Fat is also above guideline. Nontheless, because levels are low compared with most other cheeses, recommended for use as one-half of otherwise within guideline dishes.

Devondale Trim'n'Tasty Chedddar Cheese

Advertising claim: "25% reduced fat"

Food Factor	Energy	Fat	Cholest.	Sodium	Sugar	Fibre	Addit.
Labelling	1450	24.8	N.S. (.070)	.520	.1	N.S.	None
Guideline	600	2.0	.015	.120	5.0	3.75	
Conclusion	[ ]	[ ]	[ ]	[ ]	*	N.A.	*

Reductions still leave Trim'n'Tasty well above guidelines.
Not recommended.

10

Crisps and savoury snacks

As for cheeses, snack foods are generally high in energy, fat and salt. Perhaps indicating this, few snack foods display nutritional labelling. We review a cross-section of those which do.

Farmland Twin Pack Wrinkle Potato Chips -- No Added Salt

	Energy	Fat	Cholest.	Sodium	Sugar	Fibre	Addit.
Labelling	N.A.	N.A.	N.A.	.020	.7	11.9	None
Typical level	2378	39.8	N.A.				
Guideline	600	2.0	.015	.120	5.0	3.75	
Conclusion	[ ]	[ ]	N.A.	*	*	*	*

Fat and energy still markedly above guidelines, but commendable salt reduction, and much preferable to ordinary crisps. For special occasions only.

Uncle Toby's Microwave Popcorn Butter Flavour

Advertising claim: "Good for you. Has no cholesterol and is high in dietary fibre. It naturally contains complex carbohydrates and has no added sugar"

Food Factor	Energy	Fat	Cholest.	Sodium	Sugar	Fibre
Labelling	2150	29.4	0	.630	0.4	13.00
Guideline	600	2.0	.015	.120	5.0	3.75
Conclusion	[ ]	[ ]	*	[ ]	*	*

Additive Code	160(b)
Translation	Annatto
Function	Colour
Conclusion	*

However true the claimed virtues, markedly elevated in energy, fat and sodium. Not recommended.

Pringles Light BBQ Flavour Potato Chips

Advertising claim: "Cholesterol free; 1/3 less fat and salt than regular"

Food Factor	Energy	Fat	Cholest.	Sodium	Sugar	Fibre	Addit.
Labelling	2245	28.6	0	.446	N.S.	N.S.	None
Guideline	600	2.0	.015	.120	5.0	3.75	
Conclusion	[]	[]	*	[]	N.K.	N.K.	*

Despite fat and salt reductions, still well above guidelines in energy, fat and sodium. Not recommended.

New York Style Bagel Chips

Advertising claim: "No cholesterol"

Food Factor	Energy	Fat	Cholest.	Sodium	Sugar	Fibre
Labelling	1795	14.3	0	1.095	N.S.	N.S.
Guideline	600	2.0	.015	.120	5.0	3.75
Conclusion	[]	[]	*	[]	N.K.	N.A.

Additive Code	160(e)
Translation	Beta carotene
Function	Colour
Conclusion	*

Despite health atmosphere of claim 'no cholesterol', markedly elevated in energy, fat and sodium. Not recommended.

11

Soups

Conventional packaged soups can be high in fat, and are always above the guideline for sodium. For this reason, reduced fat and sodium versions are welcome — provided the reductions go far enough.

Weight Watchers Hearty Beef Instant Soup

Food Factor	Energy	Fat	Cholest.	Sodium	Sugar	Fibre
Labelling	76	.3	N.S. (.015)	.238	.2	N.S.
Guideline	600	2.0	.015	.120	5.0	3.75
Conclusion	*	*	*	[ ]	*	N.A.

Additive Code	621		415	150
Translation	MSG		Corn sugar gum	Caramel
Function	Flavour enhancer		Thickener	Colour
Conclusion	see Appendix I		*	see Appendix I

Sodium above guideline, and MSG questionable on health grounds. Not recommended.

Rosella Lite Soup -- Pumpkin

Food Factor	Energy	Fat	Cholest.	Sodium	Sugar	Fibre	Addit.
Labelling	98	.1	N.S.(O)	.255	2.4	N.S.	None
Guideline	600	2.0	.015,	.120	5.0	3.75	
Conclusion	*	*	*	[ ]	*	N.A.	*

Low fat recipe, but sodium still above guideline. Not recommended.

Rosella Lite Soup Spicy Tomato

Food Factor	Energy	Fat	Cholest.	Sodium	Sugar	Fibre	Addit.
Labelling	119	.7	N.S.(O)	.540	4.8	N.S.	None
Guideline	600	2.0	.015	.120	50	3.75	
Conclusion	*	*	*	[ ]	*	N.A.	*

Sodium well above guideline. Not recommended.

Farmland Reduced Salt Hearty Beef Single Serve Soups

Food Factor	Energy	Fat	Cholest.	Sodium	Sugar	Fibre
Labelling	104	N.S. (.05)	N.S. (<.05)	.215	<1	N.S.
Guideline	600	2.0	.015	.120	5.0	3.75
Conclusion	*	*	*	[ ]	*	N.A.

Additive Code	621	412	150	627
Translation	MSG	Guar gum	Caramel	Disodium guanylate
Function	Flavour enhancer	Thickener	Colour	Flavour enhancer
Conclusion	see Appendix I	*	see Appendix I	see Appendix I

Additive Code	631	554
Translation	Disodium inosinate	Sodium aluminosilicate
Function	Flavour enhancer	Anti-caking agent
Conclusion	see Appendix I	see Appendix I

Above guideline sodium, and some additives have been questioned on health grounds. Not recommended.

Rosella Salt Reduced Tomato Condensed Soup

Food Factor	Energy	Fat	Cholest.	Sodium	Sugar	Fibre	Addit.
Labelling	N.S. (258)	N.S. (3.4)	N.S. (<.015)	.075	5.6	N.S.(.3)	None
Guideline	600	2.0	.015	.120	5.0	3.75	
Conclusion	*	[ ]	*	*	=	N.A	*.

Despite commendable sodium level, amount of fat is likely to be above guideline. Therefore, not recommended.

Farmland Reduced Salt Cream of Chicken Single Serve Soup

Food Factor	Energy.	Fat	Cholest.	Sodium	Sugar	Fibre
Labelling	143	<1	N.S. (<.015)	.265	<1	N.S.
Guideline	600	2.0	.015	.120	5.0	3.75
Conclusion	*	*	*	[ ]	*	N.A.

Additive Code	621	412		150		627
Translation	MSG	Guar gum		Caramel		Disodium guanylate
Function	Flavour enhancer	Thickener		Colour		Flavour enhancer
Conclusion	see Appendix I	*		see Appendix I		see Appendix I

Additive Code	631		554	
Translation	Disodium inosinate		Sodium aluminosilicate	
Function	Flavour enhancer		Anti-caking agent	
Conclusion	see Appendix I		see Appendix I	

Sodium above low-salt guideline, and some additives questionable on health grounds. Not recommended.

Rosella Lite Soup -- Tasty Chicken

Food Factor	Energy	Fat	Cholest.	Sodium	Sugar	Fibre
Labelling	124	.8	N.S. (<.015)	.470	.8	N.S.
Guideline	600	2.0	.015	.120	5.0	3.75
Conclusion	*	*	*	[ ]	*	N.A.

Additive Code	1422		450	160(b)
Translation	Modified Starch		Trisodium diphosophate	Annato
Function	Thickener		Emulsifier	Colour
Conclusion	*		*	*

Elevated sodium. Hence, and despite commendable fat reduction, not recommended.

Continental Cup-a-Soup Hearty Beef -- Salt Reduced

Food Factor	Energy	Fat	Cholest.	Sodium	Sugar	Fibre
Labelling	N.S.	N.S.	N.S.	.202	N.S.	N.S.
Guideline	600	2.0	.015	.120	5.0	3.75
Conclusion	N.K.	N.K.	N.K.	[ ]	N.K.	N.K.

Additive Code	621	150	627
Translation	MSG	Caramel	Disodium guanylate
Function	Flavour enhancer	Colour	Flavour enhancer
Conclusion	see Appendix I	see Appendix I	see Appendix I

Additive Code	631
Translation	Disodium inosinate
Function	Flavour enhancer
Conclusion	see Appendix I

Sodium above guideline. Not recommended.

Rosella Salt Reduced Cream of Mushroom Soup

Food Factor	Energy	Fat	Cholest.	Sodium	Sugar	Fibre
Labelling	N.S.(22)	N.S. (3.8)	N.S.(O)	.095	.8	N.S.
Guideline	600	.2.0	.015	.120	5.0	3.75
Conclusion	*	[]	*	*	*	N.A.

Additive Code	1412		450			621
Translation	Modified Starch		Trisodium diphosphate			MSG
Function	Thickener		Emulsifier			Flavour enhancer
Conclusion	*		*			see Appendix I

Despite the commendable sodium reduction, Rosella Cream of Mushroom Soup is likely to be above guideline in fat. Therefore, not recommended.

Weight Watchers Tomato and Herb Instant Soup

Food Factor	Energy	Fat	Cholest.	Sodium	Sugar	Fibre
Labelling	75	.1	N.S. (O)	.340	.1	N.S.
Guideline	600	2.0	.015	.120	5.0	3.75
Conclusion	*	*	*	[]	*	N.A.

Additive Code	621		150	415		330
Translation	MSG		Caramel	Corn sugar gum		Citric acid
Function	Flavour enhancer		Colour	Thickener		Flavour
Conclusion	see Appendix I		see Appendix I	*		*

Above guideline sodium. Not recommended.

Farmland Reduced Salt Chicken Noodle Single Serve Soups

Food Factor	Energy	Fat	Cholest.	Sodium	Sugar	Fibre
Labelling	80	<1	N.S. (.015)	.220	<1	N.S.
Guideline	600	2.0	.015	.120	5.0	3.75
Conclusion	*	*	*	[ ]	*	N.A.

Additive Code	621	412		100		627
Translation	MSG	Guar gum		Curcumin		Disodium guanylate
Function	Flavour enhancer	Thickener		Colour		Flavour enhancer
Conclusion	see Appendix I *			*		see Appendix I

Additive Code	631	554
Translation	Disodium inosinate	Sodium aluminosilicate
Function	Flavour enhancer	Anti-caking accent
Conclusion	see Appendix I	see Appendix I

Salt above guidelines, and some additives questionable. Not recommended.

Weight Watchers Cream of Chicken Condensed Soup

Food Factor	Energy	Fat	Cholest.	Sodium	Sugar	Fibre
Labelling	102	.7	N.S. (.015)	.400	1.0	N.S.
Guideline	600	2.0	.015	.120	5.0	3.75
Conclusion	*	*	*	[ ]	*	N.A.

Additive Code	621		160(a)		101
Translation	MSG		Carotene		Riboflavin
Function	Flavour enhancer		Colour		Colour
Conclusion	see Appendix I		*		*

Above guideline sodium. Not recommended.

Alevita Mushroom Soup Mix

Advertising claim: "Meat and cholesterol free"

Food Factor	Energy	Fat	Cholest.	Sodium	Sugar	Fibre	Addit.
Labelling	126	0.7	N.S. (0)	.254	0.5	N.S.	None
Guideline	600	2.0	.015	.120	5.0	3.75	
Conclusion	*	*	*	[ ]	*	N.K.	*

Despite coommendably low fat, sodium is still elevated.
Not recommended.

Alevita Spicy Bean Soup Mix

Advertising claim: "Meat and cholesterol free"

Food Factor	Energy	Fat	Cholest.	Sodium	Sugar	Fibre	Addit.
Labelling	123	0.7	N.S. (0)	.281	0.5	N.S.	None
Guideline	600	2.0	.015	.120	5.0	3.75	
Conclusion	*	*	*	[ ]	*	N.A.	*

A generally commendable profile, but sodium is elevated. Not recommended.

Rosella Salt Reduced Pea and Ham Soup

Food Factor	Energy	Fat	Cholest.	Sodium	Sugar	Fibre
Labelling	N.S. (402)	N.S. (3.7)	N.S (<.015)	.125	N.S. (2.0)	N.S. (2.2)
Guideline	600	2.0	.015	.120	5.0	3.75
Conclusion	*	[ ]	*	=	*	N.A.

Additive Code	621	631	627
Translation	MSG	Disodium inosinate	Disodium guanylate
Function	Flavour enhancer	Flavour enhancer	Flavour enhancer
Conclusion	see Appendix I	see Appendix I	see Appendix I

Commendable sodium level, but fat likely to be above guideline Not recommended.

Rosella Salt Reduced Cream of Chicken Soup

	Energy	Fat	Cholest.	Sodium	Sugar	Fibre
Labelling	N.S.	N.S.	N.S.	.0975	N.S	N.S
	(203)	(3.6)	(<.015)		(0.7)	(<.1)
Guideline	600	2.0	.015	.120	5.0	3.75
Conclusion	*	[ ]	*	*	*	N.A.

Additive Code	621	631	627
Translation	MSG	Disodium inosinate	Disodium guanylate
Function	Flavour enhancer	Flavour enhancer	Flavour enhancer
Conclusion	see Appendix I	see Appendix I	see Appendix I

Additive Code	1422	450	160(b)
Translation	Modified Starch	Trisodium diphosphate	Annatto
Function	Thickener	Emulsifier	Colour
Conclusion	*	*	*

Fat level likely to be above guideline, and, in company with questionable additives, not recommended.

Heinz Tomato Salt Reduced Condensed Soup

Food Factor	Energy	Fat	Cholest.	Sodium	Sugar	Fibre
Labelling	126	.4	N.S(0)	.150	5.0	N.S.(.3)
Guideline	600	2.0	.015	.120	5.0	3.75
Conclusion	*	*	*	[ ]	*	N.A.

*A marked sodium reduction (down two-thirds on conventional Tomato Soup), but
still not <u>quite</u> reaching the guideline. As Heinz Salt Reduced Tomato Soup is otherwise well within guidelines for other food components, recommended for use extra diluted (i.e. with some fresh or canned no-added-salt tomatoes) so as to further reduce the sodium level.*

Hain Natural Classics Minestrone Soup Mix

Food Factor	Energy	Fat	Cholest.	Sodium	Sugar	Fibre	Addit.
Labelling	246	.53	N.S	.460	N.S.	N.S.	None
			(0)		(3.6)	(.5)	
Guideline	600	2.0	.015	.120	5.0	3.75	
Conclusion	*	*	*	[ ]	*	N.A.	*

Above guideline for sodium. Not recommended.

Massel Ultra Cube Chicken Flavoured Stock Cubes

Advertising claim: "No MSG; cholesterol free; no artificial colours, flavours or gluten"

Food Factor	Energy	Fat	Cholest.	Sodium	Sugar	Fibre
Labelling	19.97	.25	0	.065	.19	N.S(0)
Guideline	600	2.0	.015	.120	5.0	3.75
Conclusion	*	*	*	*	*	N.A.

Additive Code	627	631
Translation	Disodium guanylate	Disodium inosinate
Function	Flavour enhancer	Flavour enhancer
Conclusion	see Appendix I	see Appendix I

Because of dilution as consumed, Massel Soup in a Cube is within guidelines. But the ingredients list shows salt as the largest single ingredient. On philosophical grounds, not recommended.

Farmland Reduced Salt Single Serve Soup — Tomato

Food Factor	Energy	Fat	Cholest.	Sodium	Sugar	Fibre
Labelling	175	<1.00	N.S(0)	.215	3.0	N.S.(.3)
Guideline	600	2.0	.015	.120	5.0	3.75
Conclusion	*	*	*	[ ]	*	N.A.

Additive Code	330	331	621
Translation	Citric acid	Sodium Citrate	MSG
Function	Stabiliser	Emulsifier	Flavour enhancer
Conclusion	*	*	see Appendix I

Additive Code	412	554	100
Translation	Guar gum	Sodium alumino silicate	Curcumin
Function	Thickener	Anti-caking agent	Colour
Conclusion	*	see Appendix I	*

Additive Code	631
Translation	Disodium inosinate
Function	Flavour enhancer
Conclusion	see Appendix I

Lower salt than regular tomato soup, but still above guideline. As well, numerous of the additives have been questioned on health grounds. Not recommended.

Westbrae Natural Just Miso Soup

Food Factor	Energy	Fat	Cholest.	Sodium	Sugar	Fibre	Addit.
Labelling	61	.42	0	.300	< 1.25	N.S.	None
Guideline	600	2.0	.015	.120	5.0	3.75	
Conclusion	*	*	*	*	*	*	*

Elevated sodium. Not recommended.

Continental Cup-a-Soup Noodle Soup — Salt Reduced

Food Factor	Energy	Fat	Cholest.	Sodium	Sugar	Fibre
Labelling	N.S.(84)	N.S. (.3)	N.S. (<.015)	.182	N.S(0)	0
Guideline	600	2.0	.015	.120	5.0	3.75
Conclusion	*	*	*	[ ]	*	N.A.

Additive Code	627	631
Translation	Disodium guanylate	Disodium inosinate
Function	Flavour enhancer	Flavour enhancer
Conclusion	see Appendix I	see Appendix I

Additive Code	621	160
Translation	MSG	Beta carotene
Function	Flavour enhancer	Colour
Conclusion	see Appendix I	*

Elevated sodium, and some additives have been questioned on health grounds. Not recommended.

12

Main courses, convenience meals and packaged main course ingredients

As shown in Chapter 4 most conventional main course recipes can easily be modified to bring them within our guidelines. The same could be true of the increasing range of convenience foods available. But, as our survey shows, while fat levels are commendably being reduced, salt remains a problem.

Findus Lean Cuisine Vegetable and Pasta Mornay with Ham

Food Factor	Energy	Fat	Cholest.	Sodium	Sugar	Fibre
Labelling	373	3	N.S.	.420	<5	N.S.
Guideline	600	2.0	.015	.120	5.0	3.75
Conclusion	*	[ ]	N.K.	[ ]	=	N.A.

Additive Code		1414	469	415
Translation		Acetylated distarch phosphate	Sodium caseinate	Corn sugar gum
Function		Stabiliser	Whitener	Thickener
Conclusion		*	*	*

Elevated fat and sodium. Not recommended.

Farmland No Added Salt Baked Beans in Tomato Sauce

	Energy	Fat	Cholest.	Sodium	Sugar	Fibre
Labelling	360	0.5	0	.045	3.1	7.3
Guideline	600	2.0	.015	.120	5.0	3.75
Conclusion	*	*	*	*	*	*

Additive Code		296	150
Translation	Maize search	Malic acid	Caramel
Function	Thickener	Flavour	Colour
Conclusion		see Appendix I	

Additive Code	160(e)
Translation	Beta -8'- Apocarotenal
Function	Colour
Conclusion	*

Six-star profile. Highly recommended.

Farmland No Added Salt Spaghetti in Tomato Sauce with Cheese

Food Factor	Energy	Fat	Cholest.	Sodium	Sugar	Fibre
Labelling	280	0.9	N.S. (.002)	.050	2.0	N.S.
Guideline	600	2.0	.015	.120	5.0	3.75
Conclusion	*	*	*	*	*	N.A.

Additive Code		296		150
Translation	Maize starch	DL Malic		Caramel
Function	Thickener	Flavour		Colour
Conclusion	*	see Appendix I		*

Additive Code	160(e)
Translation	Beta -8'- apocarotenal
Function	Colour
Conclusion	*

Five star profile. Recommended.

Farmland No Added Salt Braised Steak and Onions

Food Factor	Energy	Fat	Cholest.	Sodium	Sugar	Fibre	Addit.
Labelling	505	4.5	N.S. (.021)	.048	1.6	N.S.	None
Guideline	600	2.0	.015	.120	5.0	3.75	
Conclusion	*	[]	[]	*	*	N.A.	

Elevated fat and likely elevated cholesterol.
Not recommended.

Edgell Peas and Carrots

Food Factor	Energy	Fat	Cholest.	Sodium	Sugar	Fibre	Addit.
Labelling	115	0.3	0	.207	3.0	3.8	None
Guideline	600	2.0	.015	.120	5.0	3.75	
Conclusion	*	*	*	[ ]	*	*	*

Elevated sodium. Not recommended.

Farmland Chunk Style Tuna — No Added Salt

Food Factor	Energy	Fat	Cholest.	Sodium	Sugar	Fibre	Addit.
Labelling	610	5.0	.065	.100	<1	0	None
Guideline	600	2.0	.015	.120	5.0	3.75	
Conclusion	=	[ ]	[ ]	*	*	N.A.	*

Above guidelines for fat and cholesterol. But as these are not above levels naturally occurring in tuna, recommended for use as not more than one-quarter of otherwise zero fat and cholesterol dish.

Ally No Added Salt Pink Salmon

Food Factor	Energy	Fat	Cholest.	Sodium	Sugar	Fibre	Addit.
Labelling	670	8	.090	.080	0	0	None
Guideline	600	2.0	.015	.120	5.0	3.75	
Conclusion	[ ]	[ ]	[ ]	*	*	N.A.	*

Above fat and cholesterol guidelines. But as these are not above levels naturally occurring in salmon, recommended for use as not more than one-sixth of otherwise zero fat and cholesterol dish.

Edgell No Added Salt Corn Kernels

Food Factor	Energy	Fat	Cholest.	Sodium	Sugars	Fibre	Addit.
Labelling	421	0.7	0	.002	2.7	1.6	None
Guideline	600	2.0	.015	.120	5.0	3.75	
Conclusion	*	*	*	*	*	N.A.	*

Six star profile. Recommended.

Edgell No Added Salt Whole Peeled Tomatoes

Food Factor	Energy	Fat	Cholest.	Sodium	Sugar	Fibre
Labelling	60	0.2	0	.020	2.3	.09
Guideline	600	2.0	.015	.120	5.0	3.75
Conclusion	*	*	*	*	*	N.A.

Additive Code		509	330
Translation		Calcium chloride	Citric acid
Function		Firming agent	Discolouration preventer
Conclusion		*	*

Five star profile. Recommended.

Farmland Sliced Mushrooms in Butter Sauce — No Added Salt

Food Factor	Energy	Fat	Cholest.	Sodium	Sugar	Fibre
Labelling	130	<1	<.015	.026	1.0	2.5
Guideline	600	2.0	.015	.120	5.0	3.75
Conclusion	*	*	*	*	*	N.A.

Additive Code		415	150
Translation	Modified maize starch	Corn sugar gum	Caramel
Function	Thickener	Thickener	Colour
Conclusion	*	*	see Appendix I

Five star rating. Recommended.

Farmland Green Asparagus Spears — No Added Salt

Addit.Code	Energy	Fat	Cholest.	Sodium	Sugar	Fibre
Labelling'	100	<1	0	.005	1.4	N.A.
Guideline	600	2.0	.015	.120	5.0	3.75
Conclusion	*	*	*	*	*	N.A.

Additive Code	330
Translation	Citric acid
Function	Discolouration preventer
Conclusion	*

Five star rating. Recommended.

Farmland Light Meat Chunk Tuna

Food Factor	Energy	Fat	Cholest.	Sodium	Sugar	Fibre	Addit.
Labelling	1370	26.2	.065	.430	N.S.	0	None
Guideline	600	2.0	.015	.120	5.0	3.75	
Conclusion	[ ]	[ ]	[ ]	[ ]	N.K.	N.A.	*

Several above-guideline food components. Not recommended.

Blue Lotus Foods Tofu

Food Factor	Energy	Fat	Cholest.	Sodium	Sugar	Fibre	Addit.
Labelling	370	1.4	0	.0005	<5.0	N.S.	None
Guideline	600	2.0	.015	.120	5.0	3.75	
Conclusion	*	*	*	*	*	N.A.	*

All-star profile. Recommended.

Farmland No Added Salt Red Salmon

Food Factor	Energy	Fat	Cholest.	Sodium	Sugar	Fibre	Addit.
Labelling	680	8.0	.090	.120	0	N.S.	None
Guideline	600	2.0	.015	.120	5.0	3.75	
Conclusion	[ ]	[ ]	[ ]	*	*	N.A.	*

Above guideline fat and cholesterol. But as these levels are not more than for natural salmon, recommended for use as not more than 1/3 of otherwise low fat and cholesterol recipe.

Farmland No Added Salt Australian Salmon

Food Factor	Energy	Fat	Cholest.	Sodium	Sugar	Fibre	Addit.
Labelling	790	10	.090	.050	0	0	None
Guideline	600	2.0	.015	.120	5.0	3.75	
Conclusion	[ ]	[ ]	[ ]	*	*	N.A.	*

Above guideline for fat and cholesterol. As these levels are not more than those naturally occurring in salmon, recommended for use as not more than 1/5 of otherwise low energy, fat and cholesterol dish.

Heinz Baked Beans — Salt Reduced

Food Factor	Energy	Fat	Cholest.	Sodium	Sugar	Fibre
Labelling	384	0.7	0	.268	4.4	5.00
Guideline	600	2.0	.015	.120	5.0	3.75
Conclusion	*	*	*	[ ]	*	*

Additive Code	260
Translation	Modified maize starch
Function	Thickener
Conclusion	*

A generally excellent profile. But because of the sodium level, not recommended.

Heinz Wholemeal Spaghetti in Tomato and Cheese Sauce

Advertising claim: "Five times the fibre of regular spaghetti"

Food Factor	Energy	Fat	Cholest.	Sodium	Sugar	Fibre
Labelling	273	0.7	N.S.	.405	4.5	1.60
Guideline	600	2.0	.015	.120	5.0	3.75
Conclusion	*	*	N.K.	[ ]	*	[ ]

Additive Code	330
Translation	Citric acid
Function	Stabiliser
Conclusion	*

Our calculations suggest three times rather than five times the fibre of regular (white flour) spaghetti. And, as wheat is not a markedly rich source of fibre, it is noteworthy that even the elevated fibre content of Heinz Wholemeal Spaghetti does not make it a highly significant source of fibre. As well, sodium is above guideline. Not recommended.

Edgell Country Kitchen Mexican
Pasta and Beef

Food Factor	Energy	Fat	Cholest.	Sodium	Sugar	Fibre
Labelling	481	3.0	N.S.	.699	7.1	0.15
Guideline	600	2.0	.015	.120	5.0	3.75
Conclusion	*	[]	N.K.	[]	[]	N.A.

Additive Code	1422		410
Translation	Modified starch		Corn sugar gum
Function	Thickener		Thickener
Conclusion	*		*

Additive Code	260
Translation	Acetic Acid
Function	Stabiliser
Conclusion	*

*Food components above guidelines, especially fat and
sodium. Not recommended.*

Dewcrisp Vegetables and Noodles
(for soups and casseroles)

Food Factor	Energy	Fat	Cholest.	Sodium	Sugar	Fibre
Labelling	320	<1	0	.028	1.6	N.S.
Guideline	600	2.0	.015	.120	5.0	3.75
Conclusion	*	*	*	*	*	N.A.

Additive Code	220
Translation	Sulphur dioxide
Function	Browning preventer
Conclusion	see Appendix I

*Five star rating for food components. Recommended except
for those needing to avoid the sulphur dioxide additive.*

Farmland No Added Salt Cream Style Sweet Corn

Food Factor	Energy	Fat	Cholest.	Sodium	Sugar	Fibre
Labelling	434	<1	0	.005	6.2	N.S.
Guideline	600	2.0	.015	.120	5.0	3.75
Conclusion	*	*	*	*	[ ]	N.A.

Additive Code
Translation	Cornstarch
Function	Thickener
Conclusion	*

No food component above guidelines. Recommended.

Goulburn Valley Peeled Tomatoes in Natural juice

Food Factor	Energy	Fat	Cholest.	Sodium	Sugar	Fibre
Labelling	85	N.S(0)	N.S(0)	.005	2.0	0.9
Guideline	600	2.0	.015	.120	5.0	3.75
Conclusion	*	*	*	*	*	N.A.

Additive Code   509
Translation	Calcium chloride
Function	Firming agent
Conclusion	*

More complete labelling would be a help to consumers, but
all food factors are likely to be entirely within guidelines.
Recommended

Farmland Whole Peeled Tomatoes — No Added Salt

Food Factor	Energy	Fat	Cholest.	Sodium	Sugar	Fibre
Labelling	95	<1	0	.005	2.4	0.9
Guideline	600	2.0	.015	.120	5.0	3.75
Conclusion	*	*	*	*	*	N.A.

Additive Code	509
Translation	Calcium chloride
Function	Firming agent
Conclusion	*

Straight five-star profile. Recommended.

Farmland Sliced Beetroot — No Added Salt

Food Factor	Energy	Fat	Cholest.	Sodium	Sugar	Fibre
Labelling	195	<1	0	.120	7.5	2.5
Guideline	600	2.0	.015	.120	5.0	3.75
Conclusion	*	*	*	*	[ ]	N.A.

Additive Code	260
Translation	Acetic acid
Function	Flavour
Conclusion	*

No component is above guidelines except sugars, and here the level is that naturally occurring. Recommended.

Farmland Red Kidney Beans — No Added Salt

Food Factor	Energy	Fat	Cholest.	Sodium	Sugar	Fibre.
Labelling	376	<1	0	.005	3.0	7.4
Guideline	600	2.0	.015	.120	5.0	3.75
Conclusion	*	*	*	*	*	*

Additive Code	260
Translation	Acetic acid
Function	Flavour
Conclusion	*

Straight six-star profile. Recommended.

Birdseye Crinkle Cut Oven Fries

Advertising claim: "Polyunsaturated fat; cholesterol free"

Food Factor	Energy	Fat	Cholest.	Sodium	Sugar	Febre.	Addit.
Labelling	582	4.2	Nil	.029	.7	1.3	None
Guideline'	600	2.0	.015	.120	5.0	3.75	
Conclusion	*	[]	*	*	*	N.A.	*

*Normal chips, cooked in animal fat, range in fat content from
7 to 15 per cent. On this basis, it can be shown that even
normal chips are within our cholesterol guideline. Perhaps
more relevant, however, would be the fact that Birdseye Oven
Fries are between a half and a quarter the normal fat level,
and that this is a polyunsaturated oil. Even so, this level still
remains outside guidelines. Given that zero fat chips can
easily be made — cut potatoes and toast them — despite all
the foregoing, not recommended.*

McCain Superfries — Frozen French Fried Potatoes Crinkle Cut

Advertising claim: "Cholesterol free"

Food Factor	Energy	Fat	Cholest.	Sodium	Sugar	Fibre	Addit.
Labelling	812	5.8	Neglig.	.050	0	1.3	None
Guideline	600	2.0	.015	.120	5.0	3.75	
Conclusion	[ ]	[]	*	*	*	N.A.	*

Even normal chips are low in cholesterol (see Birdseye oven Fries above), and the fat and energy levels of Superfries remain outside guidelines. Not recommended.

Steggles Frozen Chicken

Advertising claim: "More meat, less fat"

Food Factor	Energy	Fat	Cholest.	Sodium	Sugar	Fibre	Addit.
Labelling	817	13.8	.090	.070	N.S(0)	N.S.	None
Guideline	600	2.0	.015	.120	5.0	3.75	
Conclusion	[ ]	[]	*	*	*	N.A.	*

Energy, fat and cholesterol above guidelines. As is (with skin) not recommended. But without skin, and as 1/5 of otherwise zero fat, zero cholesterol recipe, recommended.

Alevita Burger Mix

Advertising claim: "Meat and cholesterol free"

Food Factor	Energy	Fat	Cholest.	Sodium	Sugar	Fibre	Addit.
Labelling	1089	11.3	0	.584	3.0	N.S.	None
Guideline	600	2.0	.015	.120	5.0	3.75	
Conclusion	[ ]	[ ]	*	[ ]	*	N.A.	*

Despite advertising claims, several food factors markedly outside guidelines.Not recommended.

Longa Life Vege-garlic Luncheon

Advertising claim: "Low salt, low cholesterol"

Food Factor	Energy	Fat	Cholest.	Sodium	Sugar	Fibre
Labelling	1125	7.6	.005	.620	<5.0	2.50
Guideline	600	2.0	.015	.120	5.0	3.75
Conclusion	[ ]	[ ]	*	[ ]	*	*

Additive Code	407	322	450
Translation	Irish moss	Lecithin	Polyphosphat.
Function	Gelling agent	Emulsifier	Buffer
Conclusion	*	*	*

Elevated fat and energy. Furthermore, sodium level is well above our guideline, as well as the official Government guideline for 'low sodium' food despite the advertising claim. Not recommended.

Tegel Turkey Hamwich

Advertising claim: "95% fat free; 40% salt reduced"

Food Factor	Energy	Fat	Cholest.	Sodium	Sugar	Fibre
Labelling	447	2.5	N.S.	.791	0.4	N.S(0)
Guideline	600	2.0	.015	.120	5.0	3.75
Conclusion	*	[ ]	N.K.	[ ]	*	N.A.

Additive Code	1422	450
Translation	Modified starch	Polyphosphates
Function	Gelling agent	Buffer
Conclusion	*	*

Additive Code	310	250
Translation	Propyl gallate	Sodium nitrite
Function	Antioxidant	Curing agent
Conclusion	see Appendix I	see Appendix I

Commendably reduced in fat (but still outside guideline); and sodium still markedly elevated. Not recommended.

Farmland Oven Fry Crumbed Fish Fillets — No Added Salt

Food Factor	Energy	Fat	Cholest.	Sodium	Sugar	Fibre
Labelling	965	16.0	N.S.	.065	<1	N.S.
Guideline	600	2.0	.015	.120	5.0	3.75
Conclusion	[ ]	[ ]	N.K.	*	*	N.A.

Additive Code	481
Translation	Sodium stearoyl lactylate
Function	Stabiliser
Conclusion	*

Above guidelines for energy and fat. Not recommended.

Plumrose off The Bone Lean Leg Ham — 20% Less Salt

Food Factor	Energy	Fat	Cholest.	Sodium	Sugar	Fibre
Labelling	546	7.0	.33	1.030	<1	0
Guideline	600	2.0	.015	.120	5.0	3.75
Conclusion	*	[ ]	[ ]	[ ]	*	N.A.

Additive Code	450	318
Translation	Sodium polyphosphate	Sodium erythorbate
Function	Stabiliser	Colour fixative
Conclusion	see Appendix I	*

Additive Code	250
Translation	Sodium nitrite
Function	Curing agent, preservative
Conclusion	see Appendix I

Several above-guideline food components, and potentially carcinogenic curing agent additive. Not recommended.

Castle Ready Leg Ham

Advertising claim: "Less salt, less fat"

Food Factor	Energy	Fat	Cholest.	Sodium	Sugar	Fibre
Labelling	466.8	4.5	.033	.846	<0.43	0
Guideline	600	2.0	.015	.120	5.0	3.75
Conclusion	*	[]	[]	[]	*	N.A.

Additive Code	450	301
Translation	Sodium polyphosphate	Sodium ascorbate
Function	Stabiliser	Colour preservative
Conclusion	see Appendix I	*

Additive Code	250
Translation	Sodium nitrite
Function	Curing agent, preservative
Conclusion	see Appendix I

Markedly less fat and sodium than average ham, but (especially sodium) still outside guidelines. As well, contains possibly carcinogenic nitrites, and nitrite-free hams are available. Not recommended.

Farmland Leg Ham — Reduced Fat, Reduced Salt

Food Factor	Energy	Fat	Cholest.	Sodium	Sugar	Fibre
Labelling	467	4.5	N.S. (.033)	.846	<1	N.S.
Guideline	600	2.0	.015	.120	5.0	3.75
Conclusion	*	[ ]	[ ]	[ ]	*	N.A.

Additive Code	450	301
Translation	Sodium polyphosphate	Sodium ascorbate
Function	Stabiliser	Colour preservative
Conclusion	see Appendix I	*

This product has the virtue of the lack of the potentially carcinogenic nitrate and nitrite curing agents in its additive list. As well, compared with orthodox ham, fat is reduced by about two-thirds. The key sticking point, however, sodium which, while reduced by one-third is still seven times the guildeline. Regretfully, not recommended.

Plumrose Lean Deli Beef

Advertising claim: "95% fat free, 20% less salt"

Food Factor	Energy	Fat	Cholest.	Sodium	Sugar	Fibre
Labelling	435	4.0	N.S. (.059)	1.030	<1	N.S(0)
Guideline	600	2.0	.015	.120	5.0	3.75
Conclusion	*	[]	[]	[]	*	N.A.

Additive Code	450	318
Translation	Sodium polyphosphate	Sodium erythorbate
Function	Stabiliser	Colour fixing accel.
Conclusion	see Appendix I	*

Additive Code	250
Translation	Sodium nitrite
Function	Curing agent, preservative
Conclusion	see Appendix I

Several above-guideline food components, as well as additives lacking generally-recognised-as-safe status. Not recommended.

Farmland Pre-Basted Turkey

Food Factor	Energy	Fat	Cholest.	Sodium	Sugar	Fibre
Labelling	750	9	N.S. (.090)	.180	N.S (<1)	N.S(0)
Guideline	600	2.0	.015	.120	5.0	3.75
Conclusion	[ ]	[ ]	[ ]	[ ]	*	N.A.

Additive Code	450	627
Translation	Potassium polyphosphate	Disodium guanylate
Function	Stabiliser	Flavour enhancer
Conclusion	see Appendix I	see Appendix I

Additive Code	631
Translation	Disodium inosinate
Function	Flavour enhancer
Conclusion	see Appendix I

Above guidelines for most food components. Not recommended

Steggles Butterball Self Basting Turkey Breast

Food Factor	Energy	Fat	Cholest.	Sodium	Sugars	Fibre	Addit.
Labelling	720	8.0	N.S. (.065)	.210	0	0	None
Guideline	600	2.0	.015	.120	5.0	3.75	
Conclusion	[ ]	[ ]	[ ]	[ ]	*	N.A.	*

Due to fat added (by injection), skinning this turkey will not necessarily reduce fat as with chicken. Sodium also added and above guidelines. Not recommended.

Farmland Ready Meals Crunchy Fish Pie

Food Factor	Energy	Fat	Cholest.	Sodium	Sugar	Fibre
Labelling	480	6.1	N.S. (.020)	.400	0	N.S.
Guideline	600	2.0	.015	.120	5.0	3.75
Conclusion	*	[ ]	=	[ ]	*	N.A.

Additive Code	1422
Translation	Acetylated distarch adipate
Function	Thickener
Conclusion	*

Elevated fat and sodium. Not recommended.

Farmland Ready Meals Curried Prawns

Food Factor	Energy	Fat	Cholest.	Sodium	Sugar	Fibre
Labelling	475	4.0	N.S.	.425	0	N.S.
Guideline	600	2.0	.015	.120	5.0	3.75
Conclusion	*	[ ]	N.K.	[ ]	*	N.A.

Additive Code	1422
Translation	Acetylated distarch adipate
Function	Thickener
Conclusion	*

Fat and sodium above guideline. Not recommended.

Farmland Ready Meals Lasagne with Bechamel Sauce

Food Factor	Energy	Fat	Cholest.	Sodium	Sugar	Fibre
Labelling	420	3.3	N.S.	.325	<1	N.S.
Guideline	600	2.0	.015	.120	5.0	3.75
Conclusion	*	[ ]	N.K.	[ ]	*	N.A.

Additive Code	1422
Translation	Acetylated distarch adipate
Function	Thickener
Conclusion	*

Above fat and sodium guidelines. Not recommended.

Findus Lean Cuisine Beef Italienne with Tagliatelle

Food Factor	Energy	Fat	Cholest.	Sodium	Sugar	Fibre
Labelling	396	2.0	N.S.	.370	13	N.S.
Guideline	600	2.0	.015	120	5.0	3.75
Conclusion	*	*	N.K.	[ ]	[ ]	N.A.

Additive Code	1422	450
Translation	Acetylated distarch adipate	Potassium poly-phosphate
Function	Thickener	Emulsifier
Conclusion	*	see Appendix I

Additive Code	150	330
Translation	Caramel	Citric acid
Function	Colour	Discolouration-preventer
Conclusion	see Appendix I	*

Above guideline sodium. Not recommended.

Findus Lean Cuisine Tuna Lasagne

Food Factor	Energy	Fat	Cholest.	Sodium	Sugar	Fibre
Labelling	399	3.0	N.S.	.360	N.S.	N.S.
Guideline	600	2.0	.015	.120	5.0	3.75
Conclusion	*	[ ]	N.K.	[ ]	N.K.	N.A.

Additive Code	1422	469
Translation	Acetylated distarch adipate	Sodium caseinate
Function	Thickener	Thickener
Conclusion	*	*

Additive Code	415
Translation	Corn sugar gum
Function	Thickener
Conclusion	*

Elevated fat and sodium. Not recommended.,

Leggo Nutrafibe Macaroni

Advertising claim: "Contains four times the fibre of regular pasta"

Food Factor	Energy	Fat	Cholest.	Sodium	Sugar	Fibre	Addit.
Labelling	1451	2.0	N.S(0)	.003	1.5	30.0	None
As consumed	464	0.6	0	.001	.48	9.6	
Guideline	600	2.0	.015	.120	5.0	3.75	
Conclusion	*	*	*	*	*	*	*

Seven star profile, and fibre indeed markedly elevated over normal wholemeal macaroni. Highly recommended.

High Plains White Hungarian Salami

Advertising claim: "Reduced fat and salt"

Food Factor	Energy	Fat	Cholest.	Sodium	Sugar	Fibre
Labelling	1000	19.5	N.S.	1.060	.8	N.S.
Guideline	600	2.0	.015	.120	5.0	3.75
Conclusion	[ ]	[ ]	N.K.	[ ]	*	N.A.

Additive Code	301	575
Translation	Vitamin C	Glucono-delta-lactone
Function	Antioxidant	Deposit preventer
Conclusion	*	*

Additive Code	250
Translation	Sodium nitrite
Function	Curing agent
Conclusion	see Appendix I

Fat and salt indeed significantly lower than for orthodox salami, but still well outside guidelines. Not recommended.

Carnation Alevita Vegetable Risotto

Advertising claim: "Designed to minimise sodium and fat without compromising flavour. No artificial colours or MSG"

Food Factor	Energy	Fat	Cholest.	Sodium	Sugar	Fibre
Labelling	446	1.8	0	.135	1.8	N.S.
Guideline	600	2.0	.015	.120	5.0	3.75
Conclusion	*	*	*	=	*	N.A.

Additive Code	1400
Translation	Maltodextrin
Function	Thickener
Conclusion	*

Although sodium level could be lower, no food factor above guidelines. Recommended.

Seakist Tuna No Added Salt

Food Factor	Energy	Fat	Cholest.	Sodium	Sugar	Fibre	Addit.
Labelling	382	1.1	N.S. (.065)	.080	.64	Nil	None
Test		4.2					
Guideline	600	2.0	.015	.120	5.0	3.75	
Conclusion	*	*	*	*	*	N.A.	*

The lower than average claimed fat level led to our test. This produced a result, for drained tuna, similar to other brands, but higher than claimed. The difference may represent batch variation or differences in method. Because both fat and cholesterol are above guideline, recommended for use but as no more than one-quarter of otherwise zero-fat, zero-cholesterol dish.

13

Sauces, stocks and dressings

Although concentrated foods, sauces, stocks and dressings can be significantly diluted by the meals with which they are consumed. Hence, our assessments were made for 10g sauce or dressing on 375g within-guideline dish (steak and salad). For stocks, dilutions were as recommended on the packaging.

Praise Light Coleslaw Dressing

Food Factor	Energy	Fat	Cholest.	Sodium	Sugar	Fibre
Labelling	1180	18.5	0	.870	26.0	N.S.
As consumed	334	1.67	.017	.102	3.17	
Guideline	600	2.0	.015	.120	5.00	3.75
Conclusion	*	*	=	*	*	N.A.

Additive Code	1422	435
Translation	Modified starch	Sorbitol esters
Function	Thickener	Emulsifier
Conclusion	*	*

Additive Code	322	471
Translation	Lecithin	Fatty acid glycerides
Function	Emulsifier	Thickener
Conclusion	*	*

Additive Code	330	160
Translation	Citric acid	Carotenoid
Function	Flavour	Colour
Conclusion	*	*

All factors within or near guidelines. Recommended.

Kraft Natural Mayonnaise

Food Factor	Energy	Fat	Cholest.	Sodium	Sugar	Fibre
Labelling	1412	27.5	N.S.(0)	.800	18.0	N.S.
As consumed	341	1.91	.016	.060	3.0	N.S.
Guideline	600	2.0	.015	.120	5.00	3.75
Conclusion	*	*	=	*	*	N.A.

Additive Code	1412	415
Translation	Modified starch	Corn sugar gum
Function	Thickener	Thickener
Conclusion	*	*

Additive Code	101	160(a)
Translation	Vitamin B2	Carotenes
Function	Colour	Colour
Conclusion	*	*

No food factor exceeds guidelines. Recommended.

Kraft Free Coleslaw Dressing

Advertising claim: "88% fat and oil free. Cholesterol free"

Food Factor	Energy	Fat	Cholest.	Sodium	Sugar	Fibre
Labelling	842	10.9	0	1.027	23.3	N.S.
As consumed	326	1.48	.016	.066	3.10	
Guideline	600	2.0	.015	.120	5.00	3.75
Conclusion	*	*	=	*	*	N.A.

Additive Code	1422	415
Translation	Modified starch	Corn sugar gum
Function	Thickener	Thickener
Conclusion	*	*

Additive Code	101	160(a)
Translation	Vitamin B2	Carotenes
Function	Colour	Colour
Conclusion	*	*

Additive Code	1400	405
Translation	Modified starch	Propulene, glycol alginate
Function	Thickener	Emulsifier
Conclusion	*	*

No factor exceeds guidelines. Recommended.

Kraft Free Mayonnaise

Advertising claim: "Cholesterol free; 87% fat free"

Food Factor	Energy	Fat	Cholest.	Sodium	Sugar	Fibre
Labelling	820	12	0	1.110	17	N.S.
As consumed	325	1.23	.016	.065	2.94	N.S.
Guideline	600	2.0	.015	.120	5.00	3.75
Conclusion	*	*	*	*	*	N.A.

Additive Code	1422	415
Translation	Modified starch	Corn sugar gum
Function	Thickener	Thickener
Conclusion	*	*

Additive Code	101	160(a)
Translation	Vitamin B2	Carotenes
Function	Colour	Colour
Conclusion	*	*

Additive Code	466
Translation	Carmellose sodium
Function	Thickener
Conclusion	*

No food factor exceeds guideline. Recommended.

Kraft Light Natural Mayonnaise

Advertising claim: "Low Cholesterol"

Food Factor	Energy	Fat	Cholest.	sodium	Sugar	Fibre
Labelling	862	12	10	1.022	18	N.S.
As consumed	326	1.51	.016	.066	2.96	N.S.
Guideline	600	2.0	.015	.120	5.0	3.75
Conclusion	*	*	=	*	*	N.A.

All food factors within guidelines. Recommended.

Rosella No Added Salt Tomato Sauce

	Energy	Fat	Cholest.	Sodium	Sugar	Fibre
Labelling	N.S.	N.S.	N.S	.017	N.S.	N.S
	(419)	(.4)	(0)		(24.5)	(1.9)
As consumed	315	1.21	.016	.040	3.73	2.26
Guideline	600	2.0	.015	.120	5.00	3.75
Conclusion	*	*	*	*	[ ]	N.A.

Additive Code	260
Translation	Acetic acid
Function	Preservative
Conclusion	*

No food factors outside guidelines. Recommended.

Farmland No Added Salt Tomato Sauce

Food Factor	Energy	Fat	Cholest.	Sodium	Sugar	Fibre
Labelling	N.S.	N.S.	N.S	.010	N.S.	N.S
	(419)	(.4)	(0)		(24.5)	(1.9)
As consumed	315	1.21	.016	.040	3.73	2.26
Guideline	600	2.0	.015	.120	5.00	3.75
Conclusion	*	*	=	*	*	N.A.

Additive Code	260
Translation	Acetic acid
Function	Preservative
Conclusion	*

No factors above guidelines. Recommended.

Alberto Culver Australia Molly McButter Butter Flavour Sprinkles

Food Factor	Energy	Fat	Cholest.	Sodium	Sugar	Fibre	Addit.
Labelling	1390	4.3	N.S.	N.S.	0	N.S.	Flavs.
Tes				4.200t			
As consumed	317	1.19	.016	.072	2.49	2.20	
Guideline	600	2.0	.015	.120	5.0	3.75	
Conclusion	*	*	=	*	*	N.A.	*

Because of the tiny amounts recommended for use*, a straight within-guideline profile. Nonetheless, because of the high intrinsic sodium level, it becomes exquisitely easy to 'overdose'. For this reason, the prudent may wish to steer clear.

*3g in 375g within-guideline steak, salad and potatoes

Kraft Free French & Herb Dressing

Advertising claim: "Cholesterol free; fat and oil free"

Food Factor	Energy	Fat	Cholest.	Sodium	Sugar	Fibre
Labelling	77	0	.0	.328	3.2	N.S.
As consumed	306	1.25	.016	.043	2.58	N.S.
Guideline	600	2.0	.015	.120	5.0	3.75
Conclusion	*	*	=	*	*	N.A.

Additive Code	330	331
Translation	Citric acid	Trisodium citrate
Function	Stabiliser	Stabiliser
Conclusion	*	*

Additive Code	410	415
Translation	Carob bean gum	Corn sugar gum
Function	Thickener	Thickener
Conclusion	*	*

Additive Code	101
Translation	Vitamin B2
Function	Colour
Conclusion	*

Food components all within guidelines. Recommended.

Kikkoman Salt Reduced Soy Sauce

Food Factor	Energy	Fat	Cholest.	Sodium	Sugar	Fibre
Labelling	288	0	N.S. (0)	3.100	9.1	N.S.
As consumed	311	1.19	.016	.120	2.73	N.S.
Guideline	600	2.0	.015	.120	5.0	3.75
Conclusion	*	*	=	=	*	N.A.

Additives Code	270
Translation	Lactic acid
Function	Preservative
Conclusion	see Appendix I

All food components within or equal to guidelines.
Recommended.

Alevita Bolognaise Style Sauce Mix

Food Factor	Energy	Fat	Cholest.	Sodium	Sugar	Fibre	Addit.
Labelling	435	4.6	0	.460	3.9	N.S.	None
Guideline	600	2.0	.015	.120	5.0	3.75	
Conclusion	*	[ ]	*	[ ]	*	N.A.	*

As consumed (50g sauce on 200g pasta), all food components
are within guidelines. Recommended.

Prue Sobers Classic Natural Pasta Sauce

Advertising claim: "No added fat, salt or sugar"

Food Factor	Energy	Fat	Cholest.	Sodium	Sugar	Fibre	Addit.
Labelling	205	0.13	0	.102	8.2	N.S.	None
Guideline	600	2.0	.015	.126	5.0	3.75	
Conclusion	*	*	*	*	*	N.A.	*

Straight five-star rating. Recommended.

Ci Bella Pasta Sauce: Primavera Style

Food Factor	Energy	Fat	Cholest.	Sodium	Sugar	Fibre	Addit.
Labelling	224	2.68	N.S(0)	.490	6.25	N.S.	None
As consumed	44	1.02	0	.104	1.25		
Guideline	600	2.0	.015	.120	5.0	3.75	
Conclusion	*	*	*	*	*	N.A.	*

Straight six-star rating as consumed. Recommended.

Kraft Free French Dressing

Advertising claim: "Cholesterol free; fat and oil free"

Food Factor	Energy	Fat	Cholest.	Sodium	Sugar	Fibre
Labelling	170	0	0	1.790	9	N.S.
As consumed	308	1.19	.016	.086	2.73	N.S.
Guideline	600	2.0	.015	.120	5.0	3.75
Conclusion	*	*	=	*	*	N.A.

Additive Code	330	331
Translation	Citric acid	Trisodium citrate
Function	Stabiliser	Stabiliser
Conclusion	*	*

Additive Code	410	415
Translation	Carob bean gum	Corn sugar gum
Function	Thickener	Thickener
Conclusion	*	*

Additive Code	101	
Translation	Vitamin B2	
Function	Colour	
Conclusion	*	

All ratings within or near guideline. Recommended.

Eta Low Salt/Low Sodium Barbecue Sauce

Food Factor	Energy	Fat	Cholest.	Sodium	Sugar	Fibre	Addit.
Labelling	800	0.6	N.S(0)	.100	47	N.S(0)	None
As consumed	325	1.21	.016	.040	3.71	2.21	
Guideline	600	2.0	.015	.120	5.00	3.75	
Conclusion	*	*	*	*	*	N. A	

No food components above guidelines. Recommended.

Kraft Cholesterol Free Polyunsaturated Mayonnaise

Advertising claim: "Low oil; Cholesterol free"

Food Factor	Energy	Fat	Cholest.	Sodium	Sugars	Fibre
Labelling	820	12	0	1.110	17	N.S(0)
As consumed	325	1.51	.016	.068	2.94	2.21
Guideline	600	2.0	.015	.120	5.00	3.75
Conclusion	*	*	=	*	*	N.A.

Additive Code	1412	415
Translation	Modified starch	Corn sugar gum
Function	Thickener	Thickener
Conclusion	*	*

Additive Code	101	160(a)
Translation	Vitamin B2	Carotenes
Function	Colour	Colour
Conclusion	*	*

Additive Code	466	
Translation	Carmellose sodium	
Function	Thickener	
Conclusion	*	

As consumed, within guidelines. Recommended.

Abundant Earth Salsa Tangy Sauce

Food Factor	Energy	Fat	Cholest.	Sodium	Sugar	Fibre	Addit.
Labelling	160	0.3	N.S(0)	.022	6.0	N.S(0)	None
As consumed	308	1.20	.016	.040	2.65	2.21	
Guideline	600	2.0	.015	.120	5.00	3.7.5	
Conclusion	*	*	=	*	*	N.A.	*

No food component above guidelines. Recommended.

Westbrae Natural Oriental Orange with Honey Dressing

Food Factor	Energy	Fat	Cholest.	Sodium	Sugar	Fibre
Labelling	266	20	0	.533	20.0	N.S(0)
As consumed	314	1.97	.016	.060	3.27	2.21
Guideline	600	2.0	.015	.120	5.00	3.75
Conclusion	*	*	=	*	*	N.A.

Additive Code	415
Translation	Xanthan gum
Function	Thickener
Conclusion	*

As consumed, no food component above guidelines.
Recommended.

Westbrae Natural Canola Oil Mayonnaise

Food Factor	Energy	Fat	Cholest.	Sodium	Sugar	Fibre	Addit.
Labelling	2838	75	N.S.(0)	.506	0	N.S.	None
As consumed	580	3.12	.016	.053	2.5	2.21	
Guideline	600	2.0	.015	.120	5.00	3.75	
Conclusion	*	[ ]	=	*	*	N.A.	*

The high fat content of Westbrae Natural Canola Oil
Mayonnaise places it above guidelines even as consumed.
Not recommended.

Norganic Imitation Bacon Bits

*Advertising claim: "No Cholesterol; no preservatives; no
animal content"*

Food Factor	Energy	Fat	Cholest.	Sodium	Sugar	Fibre
Labelling	1600	21.00.	0	2.600	10.0	N.S.
Guideline	600	2.0	.015	.120	5.0	3.75
Conclusion	[]	[]	*	[]	[]	N.A.

Additive Code	150		127
Translation	Caramel		Erythrosine
Function	Colour		Colour
Conclusion	*		see Appendix I

*This textured vegetable protein bacon substitute
unfortunately reproduces too many of conventional bacon's
above guideline features, particularly concerning sodium.
Not recommended.*

14

Desserts

Conventional desserts can be elevated in energy, fat and salt, as well as sugars.

Our survey of packaged products includes a number of new types aimed at a health-conscious market.

Farmers Union Strawberry Fruche

Advertising claim: "All natural ingredients"

Food Factor	Energy	Fat	Cholest.	Sodium	Sugar	Fibre
Labelling	464	4.0	N.S.	.037	11.9	Some
Guideline	600	2.0	.015	.120	11.40	3.75
Conclusion	*	[ ]	N.K.	*	=	N.A.

Additive Code	412
Translation	Guar gum
Function	Thickener
Conclusion	*

Fat level above guideline. Recommended for use only as not more than 50 per cent of otherwise zero fat dish.

Yoplait Light Fruit of the Forest Fruit Yoghurt

Food Factor	Energy	Fat	Cholest.	Sodium	Sugar	Fibre
Labelling	360	.07	.007	.075	17.3	0
Guideline	600	2.0	.015	.120	11.40	3.75
Conclusion	*	*	*	*	[ ]	N.A.

Additive Code	410	412	466
Translation	Carob gum	Guar gum	Carmelloso sodium
Function	Gelling agent	Thickener	Thickener
Conclusion	*	*	*

Except for sugars, a within guideline profile. Recommended for use as not more than half of otherwise low-sugars dish (e.g. with low sugar cereal).

Danone Diet Lite Strawberry Low Fat Fruit Yoghurt

Food Factor	Energy	Fat	Cholest.	Sodium	Sugar	Fibre
Labelling	190	0.13	N.S. (.007)	.066	6.6	N.S.
Guideline	600	2.0	.015	120	11.4	3.75
Conclusion	*	*	*	*	*	N.A.

Additive Code	440(a)	
Translation	Pectin	Aspartame
Function	Thickener	Sweetener
Conclusion	*	see Appendix I

All-star profile. For those not avoiding artificial sweeteners, recommended.

Peters Farm Natural Low Fat Yoghurt

Food Factor	Energy	Fat	Cholest.	Sodium	Sugar	Fibre
Labelling	248	0.17	N.S. (.007)	.088	8.11	N.S(0)
Guideline	600	2.0	.015	.120	11.4	3.75
Conclusion	*	*	*	*	*	N.A.

Additive Code	
Translation	Aspartame
Function	Sweetener
Conclusion	see Appendix I

A straight five-star profile. For those who do not wish to avoid artificial sweeteners, recommended.

Streets Calorie Control Vanilla Ice Confection

Food Factor	Energy	Fat	Cholest.	Sodium	Sugar	Fibre
Labelling(ml) 238		1.2	.0017	.025	7.1	N.S(0)
(g) 335		1.69	.002	.035	10.0	
Guideline	600	2.0	.015	.120	11.4	3.75
Conclusion	*	*	*	*	*	N.A.

Additive Code	471	407
Translation	Mono diglycerides	Carageenan
Function	Emulsifier	Stabiliser
Conclusion	*	*

Additive Code	410	466
Translation	Carob bean gum	Carmellose sodium
Function	Stabiliser	Thickener
Conclusion	*	*

Additive Code	331	102
Translation	Sodium citrates	Tartrazine
Function	Preservative	Colour
Conclusion	*	see Appendix I

Additive Code	110
Translation	Sunset Yellow
Function	Colour
Conclusion	see Appendix I

All within guideline profile, and fat markedly lower than for conventional ice-cream . Recommended (but note that two additives have been questioned on health grounds)

Peters Raspberry Sorbet and Cream

Food Factor	Energy	Fat	Cholest.	Sodium	Sugar	Fibre
Labelling(ml)	341	3.0	N.S. (<.015)	.026	9.3	N.S(0)
(g)	477	4.2	.015)	.036	13.0	(0)
Guideline	600	2.0	.015	.120	11.4	3.75
Conclusion	*	[]	*	*	=	N.A.

Additive Code	330		162
Translation	Citric acid		Beet red
Function	Preservative		Colour
Conclusion	*		*

Elevated fat level, but markedly lower than the 8–11g/100g of conventional ice-cream. Recommended for use when not more than half of otherwise zero fat dish.

Tarantos Gelato Classico Lemon

Food Factor	Energy	Fat	Cholest.	Sodium	Sugar	Fibre	Addit.
Labelling(ml)	248	0.1	N.S.(0)	.017	15	N.S(0)	None
Guideline	600	2.0	.015	.120	11.4	3.75	
Conclusion	*	*	*	*	[]	N.A.	*

Generally well within guidelines except for sugars, which are near. Recommended on special-occasion basis.

Peters Light Vanilla Milk Ice Confection

Advertising claim: "Low in fat. Contains less than 3.3% fat"

Food Factor	Energy	Fat	Cholest.	Sodium	Sugar	Fibre
Labelling(ml)	273	1.40	N.S. (<.015)	.036	8.5	N.S(0
Translation(g)	381	1.95	(<.015)	.050	11.89	(0)
Test		3.4				
Guideline	600	2.0	.015	.120	11.4	3.75
Conclusion	*	[ ]	*	*	=	N.A.

Additive Code	471	433	466
Translation	Mono diglycerides	Polysorbate	Carmellose sodium
Function	Emulsifier	Emulsifier	Thickener
Conclusion	*	*	*

Additive Code	412	110	102
Translation	Guar gum	Sunset Yellow	Tartrazine
Function	Thickener	Colour	Colour
Conclusion	*	see Appendix I	see Appendix I

Two somewhat contradictory fat levels given on the packaging. Our test result of 3.4g/l00g was close to the higher statement — a result still one-third that for conventional ice-cream. No other food factors outside guidelines. Recommended for use as 50% of otherwise zero fat dessert.

Streets Quality Favourites —
Vanilla Ice Cream Slices

Advertising claim: "100% no artificial colours or flavours"

Food Factor	Energy	Fat	Cholest.	Sodium	Sugar	Fibre
Labelling(ml)	374	4.6	N.S.	.033	8.1	N.S.
(g)	523	6.43		.046	11.3	
Guideline	600	2.0	.015	.120	11.4	3.75
Conclusion	*	[ ]	N.K.	*	*	N.A.

Additive Code	471	407	410
Translation	Mono diglycerides	Carageenan	Carob bean gum
Function	Emulsifier	Stabiliser	Stabiliser
Conclusion	*	*	*

Additive Code	412	160(b)
Translation	Guar gum	Annatto
Function	Thickener	Colour
Conclusion	*	*

Lower fat than average, but still above guideline.
Not recommended.

Cottees Apple and Peach All Natural Fruit Snack

Food Factor	Energy	Fat	Cholest.	Sodium	Sugar	Fibre	Addit.
Labelling	320	0.44	N.S(0)	.003	19.3	0.65	None
Guideline	600	2.0	.015	.120	11.4	3.75	
Conclusion	*	*	*	*	[ ]	*	

Somewhat above Guideline in sugars. Not recommended.

Farmland Pear Halves in Natural Juice

Food Factor	Energy	Fat	Cholest.	Sodium	Sugar	Fibre	Addit.
Labelling	180	<1	N.S.(0)	.006	8.7	N.S.	None
Guideline	600	2.0	.015	.120	11.4	3.75	
Conclusion	*	*	*	*	*	N.A.	*

Six star profile. Recommended.

SPC Sliced Peaches in Natural Fruit Nectar

Food Factor	Energy	Fat	Cholest.	Sodium	Sugar	Fibre	Addit.
Labelling	228	0.1	N.S.(0)	.002	11.7	1.3	None
Guideline	600	2.0	.015	.120	11.4	3.75	
Conclusion	*	*	*	*	=	N.A.	*

No food factor outside guidelines. Recommended.

Farmland Pear Halves in Light Syrup

Food Factor	Energy	Fat	Cholest.	Sodium	Sugar	Fibre	Addit.
Labelling	250	<1	N.S.(0)	.002	13.8	N.S.	None
Guideline	600	2.0	.015	.120	11.4	3.75	
Conclusion	*	*	*	*	=	N.A.	*

No food component outside guidelines. Recommended.

Sara Lee Lights Berry Topped Fruit Cheese Cake

Advertising claim: "Reduced fat, low cholesterol. Pure indulgence without the guilt"

Food Factor	Energy	Fat	Cholest.	Sodium	Sugar	Fibre
Labelling	768	9.0	.013	.079	15.0	N.S.
Guideline	600	2.0	.015	.120	11.40	3.75
Conclusion	[ ]	[ ]	*	*	[ ]	N.A.

Additive Code	477	472	270
Translation	both Glycerol	esters	Lactic acid
Function	Emulsifiers		Flavour
Conclusion	*	*	*

Additive Code	330	471	405
Translation	Citric acid	Fatty acid diglycerides	Alginate ester
Function	Flavour	Thickener	
Conclusion	*	*	*

Additive Code	407	410	415
Translation	Irish moss	Carob gum	Corn sugar gum
Function	Thickener	Thickener	Thickener
Conclusion	*	*	*

Additive Code	466
Translation	Cellulose salt
Function	Thickener
Conclusion	*

Commendable reduction in cholesterol (five-sixths) and fat (three-quarters) over typical cheesecake. However, still outside some guidelines, particularly for fat. Special occasions only.

Peters Farm Black Cherry Frozen Yoghurt

Food Factor	Energy	Fat	Cholest.	Sodium	Sugar	Fibre	Addit.
Labelling	406	2.8	N.S. (.007)	.062	12.3	N.S.	None
Guideline	600	2.0	.015	.120	11.40	3.75	
Conclusion	*	[ ]	*	*	=	N.A.	*

Fat above guideline. Not recommended.

NEW PRODUCT TYPE: INDEPENDENT LABORATORY TEST

C.C. Bottlers Limited Vitari

Advertising claim: "99% fruit and fruit juice. No cholesterol, added sugar or fat"

Food Factor	Energy	Fat	Cholest.	Sodium	Sugar	Fibre	Addit.
Labelling	N.S.	0.0	N.S(0)	N.S.	N.S.	N.S.	N.S.
Test	N.A. (<600)	0.0	N.A(0)	.038	24.3	N.A(0)	
Guideline	600	2.0	.015	.120	11.4	3.75	
Conclusion	*	*	*	*	[ ]	N.A.	

A zero-fat ice-cream substitute is a potentially important development, so we commissioned laboratory tests on key food factors. Sodium and fat levels were well within guidelines.
Despite the claim of no added sugar, the sugars test shows that Vitari in fact has a sugars level higher than any fruit, suggesting the sugar level initially present in the fruit ingredients used has been increased by concentration. Overall, recommended for special occasions.

15

Beverages

Despite health claims for such beverages as vegetable juices and mineral waters, few purchased non-milk beverage products in fact provide nutritional labelling. In this chapter we review some that do.

Orchard Fresh Orange Juice

Advertising claim: "No added sugar"

Food Factor	Energy	Fat	Cholest.	Sodium	Sugar	Fibre	Addit.
Labelling	150	<1.0	N.S(0)	.005	8.0	N.S.	None
Guideline	600	2.0	.015	.126	11.4	3.75	
Conclusion	*	*	*	*	*	N.A.	*

Within guideline profile. Recommended.

Orchard Fresh Pineapple and Orange Juice

Advertising claim: "No added sugar"

Food Factor	Energy	Fat	Cholest.	Sodium	Sugar	Fibre	Addit.
Labelling	190	<1.0	N.S(0)	<.003	10.9	N.S.	None
Guideline	600	2.0	.015	.120	11.4	3.75	
Conclusion	*	*	*	*	*	N.A.	*

Within guideline profile. Recommended.

Valencio Orange and Mango Juice

Advertising claim: "No added sugar"

Food Factor	Energy	Fat	Cholest.	Sodium	Sugar	Fibre	Addit.
Labelling	155	0	N.S.(0)	<.005	8.0	N.S.	None
Guideline	600	2.0	.015	.120	11.4	3.75	
Conclusion	*	*	*	*	*	N.A.	*

All food factors within guidelines. Recommended.

Valencio Pure Grapefruit Juice

Advertising claim: "No added sugar"

Food Factor	Energy	Fat	Cholest.	Sodium	Sugar	Fibre	Addit.
Labelling	155	0.0	N.S.(0)	<.005	6.5	N.S.	None
Guideline	600	2.0	.015	.120	11.4	3.75	
Conclusion	*	*	*	*	*	N.A.	*

Straight all-star profile. Recommended.

Valencio Dark Grape Juice

Advertising claim: "No added sugar"

Food Factor	Energy	Fat	Cholest.	Sodium	Sugar	Fibre	Addit.
Labelling	240	<1.0	N.S(0)	<.005	14.0	N.S.	None
Guideline	600	2.0	.015	.120	11.4	3.75	
Conclusion	*	*	*	*	=	N.A.	*

No food factor significantly above guideline. Recommended.

Campbells Tomato Juice

Food Factor	Energy	Fat	Cholest.	Sodium	Sugar	Fibre	Addit.
Labelling	103	.35	N.S. (0)	.301	2.8	N.S.	None
Guideline	600	2.0	.015	.120	5.00	3.75	
Conclusion	*	*	*	[ ]	*	N.A.	*

Elevated sodium. Not recommended.

Farmland No Added Salt Tomato Juice

Food Factor	Energy	Fat	Cholest.	Sodium	Sugar	Fibre
Labelling	92	<1	N.S.(0)	.004	1.8	N.S.
Guideline	600	2.0	.015	.120	5.00	3.75
Conclusion	*	*	*	*	*	N.A.

Additive Code	300
Translation	Vitamin C
Function	Browning inhibitor
Conclusion	*

Straight within guideline rating. Recommended.

Campbells V8 Vegetable Juice

Food Factor	Energy	Fat	Cholest.	Sodium	Sugar	Fibre
Labelling	85	.1	N.S.(0)	.261	2.5	N.S.
Guideline	600	2.0	.015	.120	5.00	3.75
Conclusion	*	*	*	[ ]	*	N.A.

Additive Code	260	262
Translation	Acetic acid	Sodium diacetate
Function	Stabiliser	Acidity regulator
Conclusion	*	*

Above guideline for sodium. Not recommended.

16

Confectionery

The most concentrated food consumed on its own, confectionery almost by definition cannot be within our guidelines. But because it is not seen as a staple — unlike cheese, for example — confectionery as consumed by the average Australian (that is, in strict moderation) is unlikely to affect the balance of the overall diet.

With this in mind we review a range of confectionery for which nutritional labelling is available.

Gold Crest Muesli Lites

Advertising claim: 1 "/3 less fat than our existing range. No artificial colours or preservatives"

Food Factor	Energy	Fat	Cholest.	Sodium	Sugar	Fibre
Labelling	1400	7.1	0	.035	26.2	5.3
Guideline	600	2.0	.015	.120	11.40	3.75
Conclusion	[ ]	[ ]	*	*	[ ]	*

Additive Code	422	322	330
Translation	Glycerin	Lecithin	Citric acid
Function	Humectant	Emulsifier	Food acid (preservative)
Conclusion	*	*	*

Additive Code	160(b)
Translation	Annatto
Function	colour
Conclusion	*

Outside guidelines in energy, fat and sugar, but lowest in them of the muesli bars reviewed. Markedly lower than conventional confectionery. For special occasions: recommended.

Gold Crest Yoghurt Coated Muesli Bars

Food Factor	Energy	Fat	Cholest.	Sodium	Sugar	Fibre
Labelling	1789	16.3	0	.072	36.8	3.4
Guideline	600	2.0	.015	.120	11.40	3.75
Conclusion	[ ]	[ ]	*	*	[ ]	=

Additive Code	404	1200	330
Translation	Calcium alginate	Polydextrose	Citric acid
Function	Humectant	Humectant	Food acid (preservative)

Additive Code	160(b)
Translation	Annatto
Function	colour
Conclusion	*

Elevated in a number of food components.
Not recommended.

Uncle Toby's Real Fruit Rollups

Advertising claim- "Double its weight in real fruit"

Food Factor	Energy	Fat	Cholest.	Sodium	Sugar	Fibre
Labelling	1480	4.5	0	.060	30	N.S.
Guideline	600	2.0	.015	.120	11.40	3.75
Conclusion	[ ]	[ ]	*	*	[ ]	N.A.

Additive Code	471	330	124
Translation	mono/ diglycerides	Citric acid	Ponceau 4R
Function	Emulsifier	Food acid (preservative)	colour
Conclusion	*	*	see Appendix I

*The concentration implied in 'double its weight in real fruit'
has made Uncle Toby's Real Fruit Roll Ups above guidelines
in energy, fat and sugars. But they are still lower in these
than much confectionery. For special occasions,
recommended.*

Nature Sweets Gold Label Carob Supreme Tropical Delight Block

Advertising claim: "No added sugar, artificial sweeteners, preservatives, colours, flavours or caffeine."

Food Factor	energy	Fat	Cholest.	Sodium	Sugar	Fibre
Labelling	2190	35.9	0	<.12	33	0.8
Guideline	600	2.0	.015	.120	11.40	3.7
Conclusion	[ ]	[ ]	*	*	[ ]	N.A.

Additive Code	322
Translation	Lecithin
Function	Emulsifier
Conclusion	*

Many above-guideline food components, and the vegetable oil used is palm oil, the oil highest in saturated (blood-cholesterol-raising) fat. Not recommended.

Farmland Chewy 3 Fruits Meusli Bars

Food Factor	Energy	Fat	Cholest.	Sodium	Sugar	Fibre
Labelling	1570	12	0	.180	33	2.0
Guideline	600	2.0	.015	.120	11.40	3.75
Conclusion	[ ]	[ ]	*	[ ]	[ ]	N.A.

Additive Code	322	330	160(a)
Translation	Lecithin	Citric acid	Alpha or other carotenes
Function	Emulsifier	Food acid (preservative)	Colour
Conclusion	*	*	*

Above guideline food components. Not recommended.

Uncle Toby's Topform Chunky Fruit'n-Nut Muesli Bar

Advertising claim: "Protein enriched high performance Meusli bars"

Food Factor	Energy	Fat	Cholest.	Sodium	Sugar	Fibre
Labelling	1714	13.4	0	.085	18.5	4.8
Guideline	600	2.0	.015	.120	11.40	3.75
Conclusion	[ ]	[ ]	*	*	[ ]	*

Additive Code	150	160(a)	420
Translation	Caramel	Beta carotene	Sorbitol & Glycerol
Function	Colour	Colour	Humectants
Conclusion	see Appendix I*		see Appendix I

Above guideline food components. Not recommended.

Gold Crest Chewy Choc-coated Muesli Bites — Coconut

Food Factor	Energy	Fat	Cholest.	Sodium	Sugar	Fibre
Labelling	1957	19.7	0	.066	33.1	4.6
Guideline	600	2.0	.015	.120	11.40	3.75
Conclusion	[ ]	[ ]	*	*	[ ]	*

Additive-Code	420	322	422
Translation	Sorbitol	Lecithin	Glycerine
Function	Humectant	Emulsifier	Humectant
Conclusion	see Appendix I*		*

Above guideline food components. Contains sorbitol which can be unsuitable for children. Not recommended.

Nestle NZ Canterbury Double Dipp Apricot Muesli Bar

Food Factor	Energy	Fat	Cholest.	Sodium	Sugar	Fibre
Labelling	1684	13.6	0	.110	20.3	N.S.
Guideline	600	2.0	.015	.120	11.40	3.75
Conclusion	[ ]	[ ]	*	*	[ ]	N.A.

Additive Code	322	420
Translation	Lecithin	Sorbitol
Function	Emulsifier	Humectant
Conclusion	*	see Appendix I

Above guideline food components. Sorbitol may not be suitable for young children. Not recommended.

17

Approved products

The survey in preceding chapters showed that for some food types a wide choice is available; for others the choice is limited, or, indeed, almost non-existent! We are optimistic, however, that manufacturers will move to redress the balance in these areas, just as they have for the categories which are now so much better supplied than even a year ago[R44].

In the following sections are listed food products from the survey in preceding chapters which were within guidelines for all food factors reviewed. As such, these foods are recommended for purchase.

Milks and related products
Baco Reduced Fat Luxury Chocolate Flavoured Dairy Drink

Berri Supreme Vanilla Non-diary Soy Drink

Fit 4 Ultra Filtered Low Fat Milk

Nippy's Flavoured Dairy Drinks

Pauls Go Lite Iced Coffee-Flavoured Low Fat Modified Milk

Pure Harvest Traditional Pure Soy Vanilla Drink

Sanitarium So Good Lite Low Fat Soy Drink

Skimmed Milks in general

Suncoast Shape High Calcium Low Fat Modified Milk

Suncoast Trim Reduced Fat Modified Milk

Westbrae Natural Lite Soy Drink (Plain)

Breakfast cereals
Kellogg's Puffed Wheat

Kellogg's Ready Wheats

Kellogg's Sustain

Sanitarium Granose

Sanitarium Light n Tasty Breakfast Cereal

Sanitarium Lite Bix

Sanitarium Puffed Wheat

Sanitarium Weetbix

Sanitarium Weetbix Hibran

Sanitarium Weetbix Oatbran

Uncle Toby's Fibre Plus

Uncle Toby's Multi Bran

Uncle Toby's Vitabrits

Oatbran cereals

Serves per day to meet cholesterol-reducing target[R43] are given in brackets.

Kellogg's Balance Oat Bran Flakes (3 serves/day)

Uncle Toby's Crunchy Oat Bran Breakfast Cereal (3 serves/day)

Uncle Toby's Crunchy Oat Bran Cereal with Fruit (3 serves/day)

Uncle Toby's Oat Bran (2 serves/day)

Willow Valley Crunchy Toasted Oat Bran Breakfast Cereal (2.5 serves/day)

Willow Valley Crunchy Toasted Oat Bran Breakfast Cereal with Fruit (2.5 serves/day)

Mueslis

Kellogg's Komplete Muesli Flakes

Purina Toasted Muesli Flakes

Uncle Toby's Muesli Flakes

Uncle Toby's Natural Muesli — True Swiss Formula

Breads, biscuits and cakes
Only Natural Organically Grown Rice Cakes

Riga Pritikin Bread

Ryvita No Added Salt Whole Rye Crispbread

Spreads
As consumed on salt-free bread (because of bread's energy level, all recommendations are for moderate use)

Conventional jams

Fruit spreads

Honey

Modern Health Products Natex Yeast Extract

The Island Fruit Company Australian Natural Salt Reduced Savoury Yeast Extract

Cheeses
Devondale Seven Full Flavour Cheese (only as one-fifth or less of otherwise within guideline dish)

Meadow Gold Creamed Cottage Cheese reduced Salt (only as one-half or less of otherwise within-guideline dish)

Quark Low Fat Cheese (only as one-half or less of otherwise within-guideline dish)

Crisps and savoury snacks
Preferable to conventional crisps, but still above guidelines for fat and energy — *For special occasions only*

Farmland Wrinkle Potato Chips No Added Salt

Soups
Heinz Tomato Salt Reduced Condensed Soup (only as diluted with extra fresh or canned unsalted tomatoes) .

Main courses, convenience meals and packaged main course ingredients
Alevita Bolognaise Style Sauce Mix

Alevita Vegetable Risotto

Ally No Added Salt Pink Salmon

Blue Lotus Foods Tofu

Ci Bella Pasta Sauce — Primavera Style

Edgell No Added Salt Corn Kernals

Edgell No Added Salt Whole Peeled Tomatoes

Farmland No Added Salt Australian Salmon

Farmland No Added Salt Baked Beans in Tomato sauce

Farmland No Added Salt Chunk Style Tuna

Farmland No Added Salt Cream Style Sweet Corn

Farmland No Added Salt Green Asparagus Spears

Farmland No Added Salt Red Kidney Beans

Farmland No Added Salt Red Salmon

Farmland No Added Salt Sliced Beetroot

Farmland No Added Salt Sliced Mushrooms in Butter Sauce

Farmland No Added Salt Spaghetti in Tomato Sauce with Cheese

Farmland No Added Salt Whole Peeled Tomatoes

Goulburn Valley Peeled Tomatoes

Prue Sobers Classic Natural Pasta Sauce

Seakist Tuna — No Added Salt (as no more than one-quarter of otherwise zero-fat, zero-cholesterol dish)

Steggles Frozen Chicken (skin and fat removed)

Sauces, stocks, dressings

Abundant Earth Salsa Tangy Sauce

Eta Low Salt Barbecue Sauce

Farmland No Added Salt Tomato Sauce

Kikkoman Salt Reduced Soy Sauce

Kraft Cholesterol-Free Polyunsaturated Mayonnaise

Kraft Free Coleslaw Dressing

Kraft Free French and Herb Dressing

Kraft Free French Dressing

Kraft Free Mayonnaise

Kraft Light Mayonnaise

Kraft Natural Mayonnaise

Praise Light Coleslaw Dressing

Rosella No Added Salt Tomato sauce

Westbrae Natural Organic Orange with Honey Dressing

Desserts
C.C. Bottlers Limited Vitari (as not more than one-third of otherwise within guideline dish)

Danone Diet Lite Strawberry Low Fat Fruit Yoghurt

Farmland range of Canned Fruits in Natural Juice

Farmers Union range of Fruche (as not more than 50% of otherwise within guideline dish)

Peters Farm Natural Low Fat Yoghurt

Peters Fruit Sorbets and Cream (as not more than 50% of otherwise zero fat dish)

Peters range of Light Milk Ice Confections (as not more than 50% of otherwise within guideline dish)

SPC range of Fruits in Natural Fruit Nectar

Streets range of Calorie Control Ice Confections

Tarantos Lemon Gelato Classic

Yoplait Light Yoghurts (as not more than 50% of otherwise within guideline dish)

Beverages
Brands in general of no-added sugar fruit juices

Farmland No Added Salt Tomato Juice

Confectionery
For special occasions only

Conventional Boiled sweets

Conventional Fruit drops

Conventional fruit jellies

Conventional fruit pastilles

Conventional marshmallows

Gold Crest Muesli Lites

Uncle Toby's Real Fruit Rollups

The foregoing range of branded products provides a surprisingly wide range of choice of convenient packaged foods with which to supplement the basis of the optimum diet — plenty of a wide range of fresh vegetables, and fresh fruit, moderate amounts of cereals (low sodium only) and smaller amounts of fish and lean meat.

It is hoped this approach to diet, firmly based on systematic, documented research, will assist you in selecting safer, healthier foods.

References

1. Leggett, L.M.W., and Leggett, S. M.: *The Australian Food Report* Melbourne 1989

2. Commonwealth Department of Health: Towards Better Nutrition for Australians. Canberra 1987

3.Eaton, S. B., and Konner, M.: *New England Journal of Medicine* Vol 312 pages 283–289 1985

4. Pritikin, N.: *The Pritikin Permanent Weight Loss Manual* New York 1981

5. Ornish, D., and others: Can lifestyle changes reverse coronary heart disease? *Lancet* pages 129–133 Vol. 336 1990

6. Doll, R., and Peto, R.: *The Causes of Cancer* Oxford 1981

7. Briggs, D., and Wahlqvist, M.: *Food Facts* Ringwood 1985

8. Anderson, J.W., and others: Hypolipidemic effect of high carbohydrate, high figre diets. *Metabolism* Vol 29 pages 551–558 1980

9. Hanssen, M., Marsden, J., and Norris, B.: *The New Additive Code Breaker* Melbourne 1989

APPENDIX I: Additives with health implications

Additive Number	Additive Name	Suggested Health Effect
102	Tartrazine	Allergic reactions in already over-active children, some asthmatics and some aspirin-intolerant people
110	Sunset Yellow	Allergic reactions in aspirin-intolerant people
124	Ponceau 4R	Allergic reactions in some aspirin sensitive and some asthmatic people
127	Erythrosine	Carcinogenic to animals; can cause allergies reactions
211	Sodium benzoate	Allergic reactions in some asthmatics, aspirin-sensitive people and urticaria sufferers
220	Sulphur dioxide	Possible risk to people with impaired liver or kidneys; can cause asthma attacks in asthmatics

250 & 251	Sodium Nitrite	Potentially carcinogenic; can produce breathing problems
270	Lactic acid	Can cause problems for babies
281	Sodium propionate	Link with migraines
296	DL — Malic acid	Should not be given to infants and young children. (Not known if they can digest it)
310	Proplyl gallate	Reactions in asthmatics and apsirin-sensitive people. Must not be given to children
320	Butylated hydroxyanisole	Possible carcinogen. Must not be given to children
339	Sodium phosphate monobasic	High intakes may upset calcium/phosphorous metabolism
420	Sorbitol and sorbitol syrup	Can cause minor stomach and abdominal problems. Should not be given to children

Additive Number	Additive Name	Suggested Health Effect
450	The pyrophosphates	High intakes may upset calcium/phosphorous metabolism
508	Postassium chloride	Associated with gastric ulcers (high doses). Should not be given to children
554	Sodium aluminosilicate	Aluminium is associated with nerve damage and Alzheimer's disease
621	MSG	Can cause discomfort (Chinese Restaurant Syndrome). May be associated with brain damage
627	Disodium guanylate	No adverse effects known, but prohibited for use in foods for children and infants
631	Disodium inosinate	No adverse effects known, but prohibited for use in foods for children and infants
	Aspartame	Adverse effects only for sufferers of rare genetic disorder phenylketonuria (affects one in 16,000 people)